Surgical Pathology

Ahmad Altaleb
Editor

Surgical Pathology

A Practical Guide for Non-Pathologist

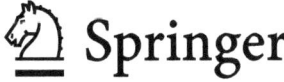 Springer

Editor
Ahmad Altaleb
Histopathology Department
Mubarak Alkabeer Hospital
Jabriya
Kuwait

ISBN 978-3-030-53689-3   ISBN 978-3-030-53690-9   (eBook)
https://doi.org/10.1007/978-3-030-53690-9

This Springer imprint is published by the registered company Springer Nature Switzerland AG
The registered company address is: Gewerbestrasse 11, 6330 Cham, Switzerland

Images are among the strongest stimuli to the imagination. This is why microscopic observations have been so fertile in biomedical science. Surgical pathologists spend a great part of their lives peering through a microscope, which activity may be called "diagnostic recognition." They try to match the image of what they see with a preexisting image stored, along with a huge number of others, in the memory

Frank González-Crussí, MD.

González-Crussí F. A quick sketch of the surgical pathologist, from nature. Semin Diagn Pathol. 2008;25(3):130–5.

This work is dedicated with great appreciation to my parents, wife, children, and to my country Kuwait.

Foreword

To the public and even the health-care professionals, pathology is like a black box where specimen went in and reports come out in a few days. Nobody knows what happened in the black box and people only care when the report delayed or when the error occurred. Physicians and surgeons often puzzled with some of the terms used in the report. What cribriform, basaloid, alveolar, hobnail, and herringbone mean to the patient? Why does error occur in pathology? The old proverb says, "Difference in profession makes one feel worlds apart." The intention of this *Notebook of Surgical Pathology* is to open that black box and bridge that knowledge gap between pathology and other health-care professions.

This book represents a joint effort of education leaders in both pathology and surgery. It covers a wide range of topics from describing the technical process of pathology and the commonly used terms in pathology reports to explaining the limitations of the pathology as a subjective specialty and different stages of specimen handling and processing that could cause error in the final diagnosis. I am particularly impressed with the figures and diagrams that help the authors to explain a complicated process in a visual, simplistic way. In my opinion, this book will be an excellent reference not only for practicing physicians but also, probably more importantly, for medical students and first-year pathology residents to gain a quick understanding of the basics of pathology laboratory.

I applaud the efforts made by the authors and the novel concept of this book. I look forward to seeing the final print in the medical literature.

Zu-hua Gao
Department of Pathology
McGill University Faculty of Medicine
Montreal, QC, Canada
April 5, 2020

Preface

This book makes no claims to be a textbook of surgical pathology as many aspects of this specialty are not included. It is rather a collection of summaries in the form of infographics/mind maps and illustrations, in an attempt to simplify major concepts of surgical pathology through high-yield fact pages designed for the busy surgeon and health-care professionals. To achieve this goal, it was deliberate to reduce the text and rely more on visual representations in order to communicate information and knowledge "at glance."

The idea to prepare this work evolved from my observations over the years. I have noticed that the vast majority of surgical colleagues including trainees or residents have no clue about the pathologists' task and the practical aspects inside the pathology laboratory.

Focusing solely on the aforementioned issue, I decided to abandon discussing pathologic entities and histologic features of diseases, as these can be learned from major textbooks like *Rosai and Ackerman's* or *Sternberg's Diagnostic Surgical Pathology*.

So, the main purpose of this book is to provide a succinct background of practical surgical pathology, its important terminology, concepts, and some technical aspects. It is also intended to bridge the gaps between pathology and surgery as well as other health-care professionals.

I hope you enjoy this book and find it very useful in your practice.

Kuwait   Ahmad Altaleb

Acknowledgments

I owe a great debt to many individuals for their inspiration and support.

I acknowledge my outstanding pathologist, teacher, and colleague, Dr. Issam Francis, who inspired me during my training and was a source of consistent motivation to learn pathology. I am grateful to Dr. Sundus Hussein, my previous pathology program director, for her continuous support and encouragement. Also, I would like to thank all senior and junior pathologists who helped me one day to learn pathology.

It is important to acknowledge the assistance of Springer Nature associate editor Mr. Wyndham Hacket Pain for his most helpful assistance from the first contact with him, and all Springer Nature staff who were very cooperative and available whenever needed.

Contents

Contributors

Khaled Alyaqout Surgical Department, Jaber Al-Ahmad Hospital, South Surra, Kuwait

Jurre Blom Maastricht University, Maastricht, Netherlands

Nicolas Kozakowski Department of Pathology, Medical University of Vienna, Vienna, Austria

Ali Lairy Surgical Department, Mubarak Al Kabeer Hospital, Ministry of Health, Jabriya, Kuwait

Ali Lari Department of Orthopedics, Jaber Al-Ahmad Hospital, South Surra, Kuwait

Eisa Lari Surgical Department, Jaber Al-Ahmad Hospital, South Surra, Kuwait

João Palma Pathology Department, Hospital Vila Franca de Xira, Lisbon, Portugal

Esperança Ussene Pathology Department, Hospital Vila Franca de Xira, Lisbon, Portugal

Part I
Introduction

The Role of Surgical Pathologist: A Surgeon's Perspective

Eisa Lari, Ali Lari, and Khaled Alyaqout

Objective

- Learn the importance of surgical pathologist's role pre-, intra-, and postoperatively, from surgeons' point of view.

Introduction

A plethora of clinical diagnoses remains tethered to the definitive diagnosis confirmed by the pathologist. In practice, a high index of clinical suspicion cannot always allow for the procession of treatment, especially in cases of suspected malignancy. Thus a surgeon's ability to clinically confirm a pathologic diagnosis is inevitably limited. With rapid advancement in healthcare and patient expectations, assigning a diagnosis of malignancy based on suspicion is no longer mainstay (Connolly et al. 2003). Various types of pathologists exist, each specialized in dealing with different samples.

As such, the role of the pathologist in surgery is emphasized. A prominent aspect of determining management relies upon the pathologist. Whether assessing gross specimens or examination by microscope. Various techniques have been adopted to aid in diagnosis, including frozen sections and permanent sections. The surgeon relies on the pathologist to grant insight on tissue characteristics. Even if the tissue itself looks grossly abnormal or "malignant," appropriate analysis of the tissue structure is essential. The pathologist may examine the tissue grossly (macroscopically).

E. Lari · K. Alyaqout (✉)
Surgical Department, Jaber Al-Ahmad Hospital, South Surra, Kuwait

A. Lari
Department of Orthopedics, Jaber Al-Ahmad Hospital, South Surra, Kuwait

© The Editor(s) (if applicable) and The Author(s), under exclusive license to Springer Nature Switzerland AG 2021
A. Altaleb (ed.), *Surgical Pathology*,
https://doi.org/10.1007/978-3-030-53690-9_1

Tissue sections may be examined under a light microscope in more detail. Different techniques are carried out to provide further information including special/immuno-histochemical staining and molecular testing.

Preoperative Input

The pathologist is present in multidisciplinary team (MDT) meetings. As a display of more comprehensive communication, it may prove more fruitful than sending a report with subspecialized "jargon" (Carter 1997). Underscoring the necessity of ensuring that the scientific language used is understood by both parties. Furthermore, surgeons and pathologists must work in harmony, a clear multidisciplinary collaboration between both specialties is time-efficient and acts in the best interest of the patient. In an MDT meeting, input onto tissue characteristics and how they respond to different therapy is vital (see Chap. 24).

The pathologist's input is essential and highlighted in the diagnosis of breast cancer. Pathology is one of the pillars in the triple assessment in diagnosis of breast cancer; with clinical examination and radiology occupying the other two roles. For example, a suspicious lesion is detected clinically and radiographically. However, proceeding with surgery is likely unwarranted based on suspicion alone. Histological type, features of malignancy, degree of invasion, receptor status, and grade of differentiation are a few examples that can be attained by the pathologist (Leong and Zhuang 2011).

On a biopsy, immunohistochemical analysis can be performed to identify immunohistochemical biomarkers such as estrogen receptor, progesterone receptor, and Her2 receptor status. These can alter the management and even determine whether the lesion is best treated with surgery, chemotherapy, hormonal therapy, or a combination therapy. Therapeutic application of this data may even alter prognosis (Leong and Zhuang 2011).

Intraoperative Input

The pathologist can be present intraoperatively to grossly examine tissue or be sent the sample via personnel or tube systems. It is essential that efficient communication occurs between the surgeon and the pathologist in order to avoid errors and optimize management.

There is no doubt that the intraoperative role of the pathologists is essential in many cases (see Chaps. 12–14).

Postoperative Input

Postoperatively, analysis of tissue guides further management. It can give insight into whether excision margins were clear or require re-excision.

Different consultations are made by different surgical subspecialties. A general surgeon may request information regarding lymph nodes status in breast cancer. Whereas a plastic surgeon would request surgical excision margins taken during excision of a squamous cell carcinoma of the skin. The task of the pathologist may often revolve around malignancy.

The pathologist plays a role in determining pathogenesis, its clinical correlation, behavior of neoplasm, and estimate prognosis accordingly. The surgeon can therefore pragmatically approach the diagnosis, and more accurately assess further management, or to an extent, estimate prognosis.

References

Connolly JL, Schnitt SJ, Wang HH, et al. Role of the surgical pathologist in the diagnosis and management of the cancer patient. In: Kufe DW, Pollock RE, Weichselbaum RR, et al., editors. Holland-Frei cancer medicine. 6th ed. Hamilton: BC Decker; 2003.

Carter D. Surgical pathology at Johns Hopkins. In: Rosai J, editor. Guiding the surgeon's hand: the history of American surgical pathology. Washington, DC: American Registry of Pathology; 1997. p. 23–39.

Leong AS-Y, Zhuang Z. The changing role of pathology in breast cancer diagnosis and treatment. Pathobiology. 2011;78(2):99–114. https://doi.org/10.1159/000292644.

Esperança Ussene

Objective

- Learn the main differences between the diagnostic role of histopathology and cytopathology and the type of samples they utilize for diagnosis

E. Ussene (✉)
Pathology Department, Hospital Vila Franca de Xira, Lisbon, Portugal

HISTOPATHOLOGY & CYTOPATHOLOGY

HISTOPATHOLOGY

- Tissues are obtained through biopsies (incisional/excisional) or surgical specimens

- This tissue goes through a series of processing until getting ready to be examined under the microscope Histological sections provide the pathologist with microscopic details of the tissues and organs of the human body

📖 DEFINITION

- It is a branch of pathology that studies and interprets disease in a tissue section

- It is a relatively longer and more expensive technique

HISTOPATHOLOGY VS. CYTOPATHOLOGY

📖 DEFINITION

- It is the branch of pathology that studies diseases through observation and interpretation of changes that occur in cells

- That is, the pathologist does not observe the architecture of the tissue as a whole, but only the characteristics of the cells

CELL BLOCK

Refers to the inclusion in paraffin blocks of cytology samples that can be cut and stained by the same methods used for histopathology. This technique provides additional information on tissue architecture and can be used to make ancillary techniques such as immunocytochemistry and molecular techniques

CYTOPATHOLOGY

- The cells may be exfoliated from epithelial surfaces and cavities or removed from various organs and tissues (by fine needle aspiration)

- It is a relatively faster and cheaper technique, allowing quickly differential diagnosis between benign and malignant lesions

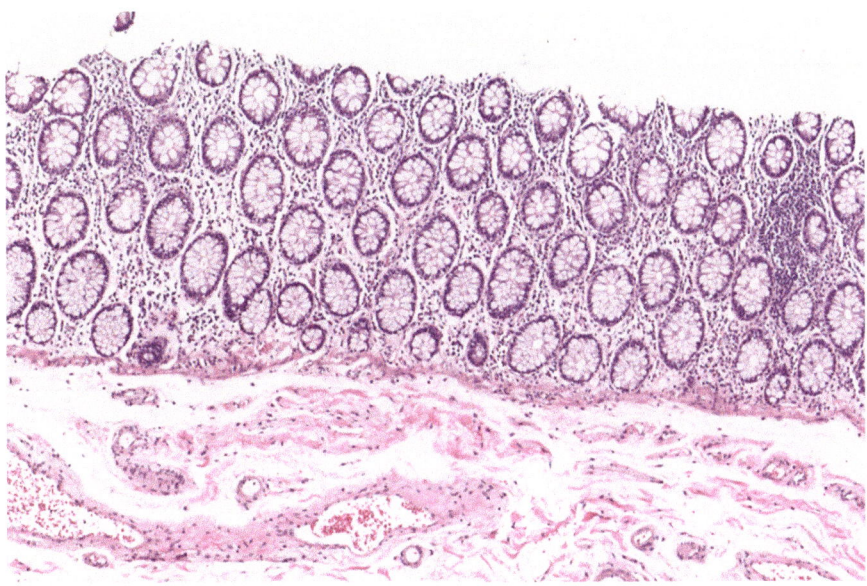

Fig. 2.1 Histology section of the normal colonic mucosa and part of the submucosa. The architecture of tissue and the features of its layers can be studied from this power of magnification. Hematoxylin and eosin stain (H&E stain), ×100

Fig. 2.2 Histology section of the normal thyroid gland. Hematoxylin and eosin stain (H&E stain), ×100

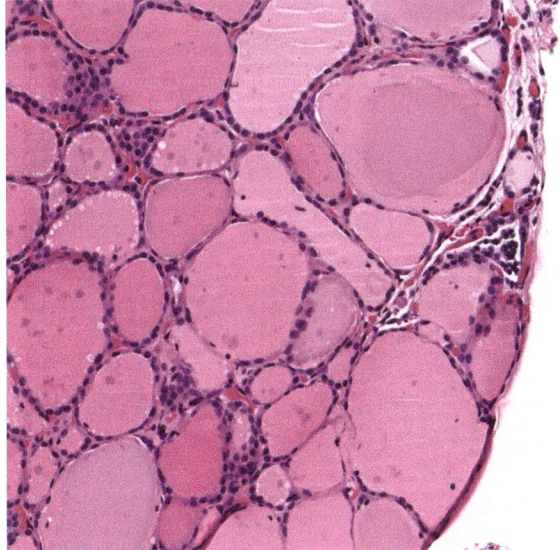

Fig. 2.3 Pap smear of uterine cervix reveals benign squamous epithelial cells. Also seen are scattered inflammatory cells. The characteristics of cells can be studied in detail. However, it is not possible to study the tissue architecture. Papanicolaou stain, ×200

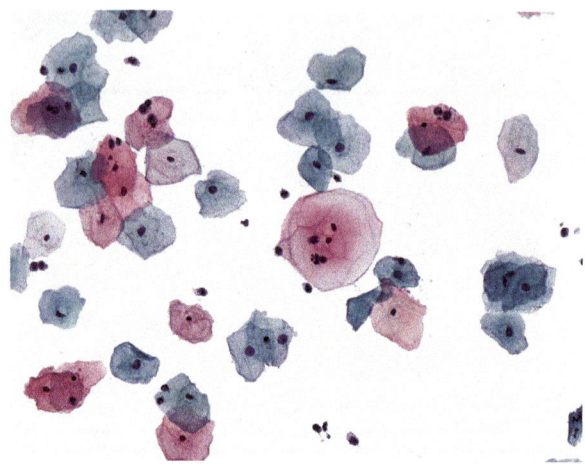

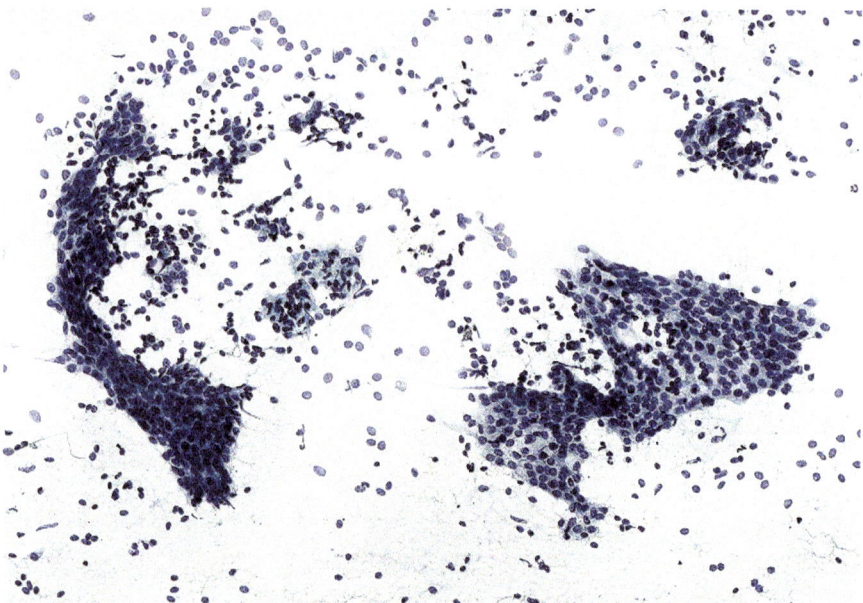

Fig. 2.4 Fine needle aspiration (FNA) smear of breast fibroadenoma shows groups of cells and tissue fragments. Notice the numerous dispersed cells in the background. Diff-Quick stain, ×100

Further Reading

Al-Abbadi M. Basics of cytology. Avicenna J Med. 2011;1(1):18.

Chandra A, Nhsft ST, Maddox A, Hertfordshire W, Nhs H. Tissue pathways for diagnostic cytopa-thology October 2019. 2019;(October):1–33.

Lester SC. Manual of surgical pathology: expert consult. 2010. 592 p.

Sharma R. Role of cell block in diagnostics—a new paradigm in cancer diagnosis. Int Clin Pathol J. 2015;1(5):113–8.

Syed S. Histopathology specimens. J Pak Med Assoc. 1992;42:51.

Part II

The Surgical Pathology Report

The Surgical Pathology Request Form, What Is Mandatory To Fill-In?

3

Esperança Ussene

Objective

- Learn the necessary data that should be provided to the pathologist for a proper clinicopathologic correlation and establishing an accurate diagnosis.

E. Ussene (✉)
Pathology Department, Hospital Vila Franca de Xira, Lisbon, Portugal

A. Altaleb (ed.), *Surgical Pathology*,
https://doi.org/10.1007/978-3-030-53690-9_3

15

THE SURGICAL PATHOLOGY REQUEST FORM

A completed request form must accompany the patient sample. It MUST contain the following correct information:

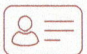

MANDATORY:
PATIENT IDENTIFICATION

- Patient's full name
- Date of birth
- Hospital number
- Patient's address

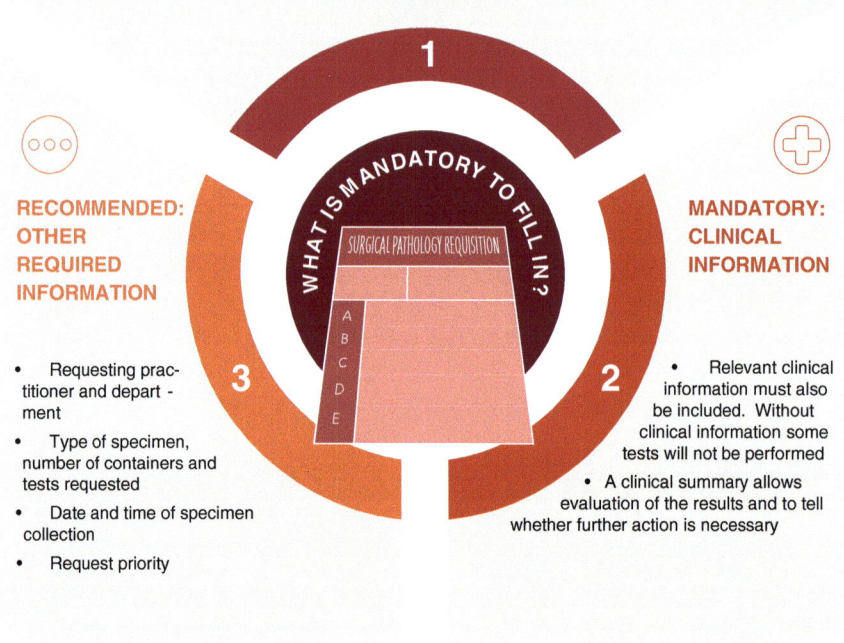

RECOMMENDED:
OTHER
REQUIRED
INFORMATION

- Requesting prac-
  titioner and depart -
  ment
- Type of specimen,
  number of containers and
  tests requested
- Date and time of specimen
  collection
- Request priority

MANDATORY:
CLINICAL
INFORMATION

- Relevant clinical
  information must also
  be included. Without
  clinical information some
  tests will not be performed
- A clinical summary allows
  evaluation of the results and to tell
  whether further action is necessary

Further Reading

Bailey J, Jennings A, Parapia L. Change of pathology request forms can reduce unwanted requests and tests. J Clin Pathol. 2005;58(8):853–5.

Singh H, Charaya N, Poonia M, Kaur Sidhu S, Singh Sihmar S. Biopsy—a vision of life. Int J Contemp Med Res [Internet] 2016;3(6):2454–7379. www.ijcmr.com.

The Surgical Pathology Report Simplified

4

Ahmad Altaleb

Objective

- Learn the structure of the surgical pathology report and the essential components of it.

The surgical pathology report primarily serves as a communication method between the pathologist and the clinician and sometimes among the pathologists themselves.

It has specific components that document, describe, and elucidate the macroscopic and the microscopic pathologic changes present in the specimen, ancillary studies performed, and the final diagnosis (Table 4.1).

The report should contain all the information to which the pathologist has access, that is, necessary to plan the patient management. This information varies according to tumor origin, type, and staging system employed. Furthermore, the reporting style might show some variation among different institutions.

Many attempts have been made to standardize the surgical pathology report and several reporting templates and protocols were generated for this purpose (Fig. 4.1).

Standardization would ensure completeness of the report and avoiding omission of essential information that contribute to patient management plan and prognostication. It also helps with quality assurance and clinical research purposes.

Surgical pathology reports may also contain educational comments, opinions, or recommendations for the treating clinician that would help in optimizing patient care. This is usually mentioned under the "comment" section.

Finally, reports should be issued promptly to avoid any delay in patient care (thus uselessly adding to the cost of medical care, leading to error, confusion, and prolonged anxiety in patients who are often already distressed).

A. Altaleb (✉)
Histopathology Department, Mubarak Alkabeer Hospital, Jabriya, Kuwait

A. Altaleb (ed.), *Surgical Pathology*,
https://doi.org/10.1007/978-3-030-53690-9_4

Table 4.1 The components of the surgical pathology report

Report component	Items	
Patient demographics	Name, age, date of birth, gender, address	
Clinical data	Pertinent clinical information	
Gross description	Number and type of submitted specimen(s), pathologic changes, characteristics of the lesion, distance from the surgical margin, etc. Submitted sections/cassettes summary	
Microscopic description	Tumor type, grade, stage, nonneoplastic changes, ancillary studies (e.g., immunohistochemistry, molecular)	
Diagnosis	Tumor type, grade, stage, other relevant major findings	
Comments	(If applicable) expressing pathologist's opinion/concern or advice	
Addendum/amendments	(If applicable) any added result of pending tests or any change in the diagnosis after issuing of the final report	

Surgical pathology report

Name:
Age/Sex/DOB
Med Record #:
Patient #:

Requesting
Physician:
Date of Procedure:
Date Received:
Date of Report:

FINAL DIAGNOSIS

THYROID, TOTAL THYROIDECTOMY-

Papillary thyroid carcinoma, conventional type(1·7cm), right lobe

No capsular or angiolymphatic invasion

Margin is free of carcinoma

Pathologic stage pT1bNx

Background of focal lymphocytic thyroiditis

Surgical Pathology Cancer Case Summary (Synoptic) Report

This substitutes the 'microscopic description' section
Here you get most of the details you are looking for!

Procedure
Total thyroidectomy

Tumor Focality
Unifocal
Tumor Site
Right lobe
Tumor Size
Greatest dimension (centimeters): 1·7 cm
    Additional dimensions (centimeters): 1·5 x 0·9 cm

Histologic Type
Papillary carcinoma, classic (usual, conventional)
Margins
Uninvolved by carcinoma
Angioinvasion (Vascular Invasion)
 Not identified

Fig. 4.1   Sample surgical pathology report using a Cancer Reporting Protocol Template

Lymphatic Invasion
 Not identified

Extrathyroidal Extension
 Not identified

Primary Tumor (pT)
pT1b: Tumor >1 cm but ≤ 2 cm in greatest dimension, limited to the
           thyroid

Regional Lymph Nodes (pN)
pNX: Regional lymph nodes cannot be assessed

Additional Pathologic Findings
Focal lymphocytic thyroiditis

COMMENT

 Pending Biomarkers result· *An addendum will be issued·*

> Hold on! More investigations are being carried out!

CLINICAL HISTORY:

Papillary carcinoma

GROSS DESCRIPTION:

Received in formalin, labeled with the patient's name, unit number, and "thyroid," is an 85-gram total thyroidectomy specimen consisting of right lobe (6 x 3·5 x 3 cm), left lobe (8 x 5 x 4 cm), and isthmus (2 x 1·4 x 1cm)· There is a 1·7x1·5x0·9cm ovoid white to tan firm tumor with a finely granular appearance present in the right lobe· The tumor is poorly circumscribed and grossly does not invade into the adjacent capsule (0·3cm from the inked resection margin)· The remainder of the parenchyma is red/brown and homogeneous without other lesions noted·
Cassettes #1-2: Tumor with inked thyroid excision margin, 2 frags, entire specimen submitted·
Cassettes #3-7: Remainder of tumor including the entire tumor capsule, 1 to 3 frags each, entire specimen submitted·

> No more tissue of this type can be submitted.

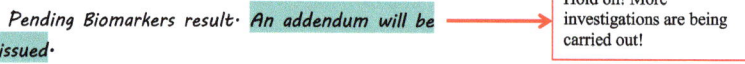

Fig. 4.1 (continued)

Cassettes #8-9: Right lobe, away from tumor, 2 frags, **representative sections submitted·**

Cassette #10: Isthmus, 1 frag, representative sections submitted·

Additional tissue of this type could be submitted if required.

Cassettes #11-12: Representative .... *section of left lobe, 2 frags, representative sections submitted·*

Report Electronically Signed by:
Surgical Pathologist

Fig. 4.1 (continued)

Further Reading

Cancer Protocol Templates [Internet]. College of American Pathologists. 2010. [Cited 2020 Mar 10]. https://www.cap.org/protocols-and-guidelines/cancer-reporting-tools/cancer-protocol-templates.

Connolly JL, Schnitt SJ, Wang HH, et al. Role of the surgical pathologist in the diagnosis and management of the cancer patient. In: Kufe DW, Pollock RE, Weichselbaum RR, et al., editors. Holland-Frei cancer medicine. 6th ed. Hamilton: BC Decker; 2003.

Lester SC. Manual of surgical pathology: expert consult. 3rd ed. Philadelphia: Elsevier/Saunders; 2010.

Weidner N. Modern surgical pathology. Philadelphia: Saunders/Elsevier; 2009.

Clarifying Jargon in Pathology Reports

5

Ahmad Altaleb and Nicolas Kozakowski

Objective

- Learn and understand some frequently used terminology in pathologist's language and the hidden meanings behind them.

A. Altaleb (✉)
Histopathology Department, Mubarak Alkabeer Hospital, Jabriya, Kuwait

N. Kozakowski
Department of Pathology, Medical University of Vienna, Vienna, Austria
e-mail: nicolas.kozakowski@meduniwien.ac.at

25

(a) Terminology used to describe cellular morphology

CLEAR CELL TUMORS

DEFINITIONS

- A tumor formed by proliferation of clear cells.

- Clear cells: are cells which show clear 'transparent' cytoplasm – seen as white (by H&E).

- The cytoplasmic contents (lipids / glycogen) impart this appearance on H&E stained sections.

CONSIDERATIONS

1. A long list of tumors enter the differential diagnosis.

2. Tumor site and 2° accompanying features can help to narrow down differential diagnosis.

3. Immunohistochemical stains are of great help in case of metastatic tumors.

NOTE: Many tumors can show clear cell change (focally) – this is different than clear cell tumors.

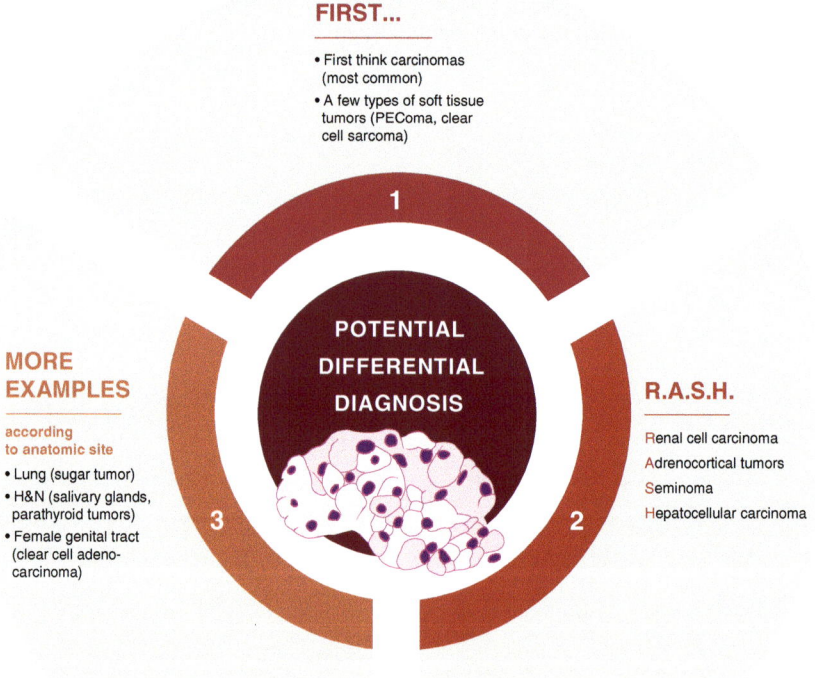

FIRST...

- First think carcinomas (most common)
- A few types of soft tissue tumors (PEComa, clear cell sarcoma)

1

POTENTIAL DIFFERENTIAL DIAGNOSIS

MORE EXAMPLES

according to anatomic site

- Lung (sugar tumor)
- H&N (salivary glands, parathyroid tumors)
- Female genital tract (clear cell adenocarcinoma)

3

2

R.A.S.H.

Renal cell carcinoma
Adrenocortical tumors
Seminoma
Hepatocellular carcinoma

EPITHELIOID CELL TUMORS
(EPITHELIOID MORPHOLOGY)

DEFINITIONS

Epithelioid → epithelial – like (resembling epithelium)
Large polygonal cells with abundant cytoplasm & round/ovoid nuclei

CAN BE BROADLY CLASSIFIED INTO

IMMUNOSTAINS

1

- True epithelial origin (i.e carcinomas – primary or secondary)

Epithelioid malignancies are often carcinomas

- Soft tissue origin or sarcomas (e.g. epithelioid sarcoma, epithelioid GIST, alveolar soft part sarcoma)

- Melanomas
- Mesotheliomas

Can acquire epithilioid morphology

2

Immunostains could be helpful in determining the origin of tumors with epithelioid morphology

Examples

- Pan-cytokeratin (pan-CK): positive in carcinomas

- S100, HMB45 and Melan A: positive in melanomas

SMALL ROUND (BLUE) CELL TUMORS

DEFINITIONS

- A group of aggressive malignant neoplasms/tumors composed of relatively small and monotonous undifferentiated cells with high nuclear-cytoplasmic ratio.

- They appear blue by H&E stain owing to the scant cytoplasm and high enlarged nucleus (which is blue (basophilic)).

CONSIDERATIONS

Since they are poorly differentiated/un - differentiated →more difficult to render a diagnosis.

The origin of these tumors can be:

1. Hematolymphoid (e.g. lymphomas)
2. Soft tissue (sarcomas)
3. Epithelial (small cell carcinomas)

FINAL DIAGNOSIS

Histomorphology + Immunohistochemis - try + Flow cytometry (for lymphomas) + Molecular/Cytogenetic testing.

PEDIATRIC SRCT

A Lymphomas
- Lymphoblastic lymphoma

B Sarcomas (Blastomas)
- Ewing sarcoma
- Rhabdomyo sarcoma
- Wilms tumor (Nephroblastoma)
- Neuroblastoma
- Medulloblastoma
- Retinoblastoma
- Hepatoblastoma

ADULT SRCT

A Non-Hodgkin Lymphoma

B Carcinoma
- Small Cell Carcinoma
- Merkel Cell Carcinoma (skin malignancy)

C Sarcomas
- Synovial Sarcoma
- Desmoblastic Small Round Cell Tumor (DSRCT)
- Myxoid/Round Cell Liposarcoma
- Small Cell Osteosarcoma
- Mesenchymal Chondrosarcoma
- Olfactory Neuroblastoma

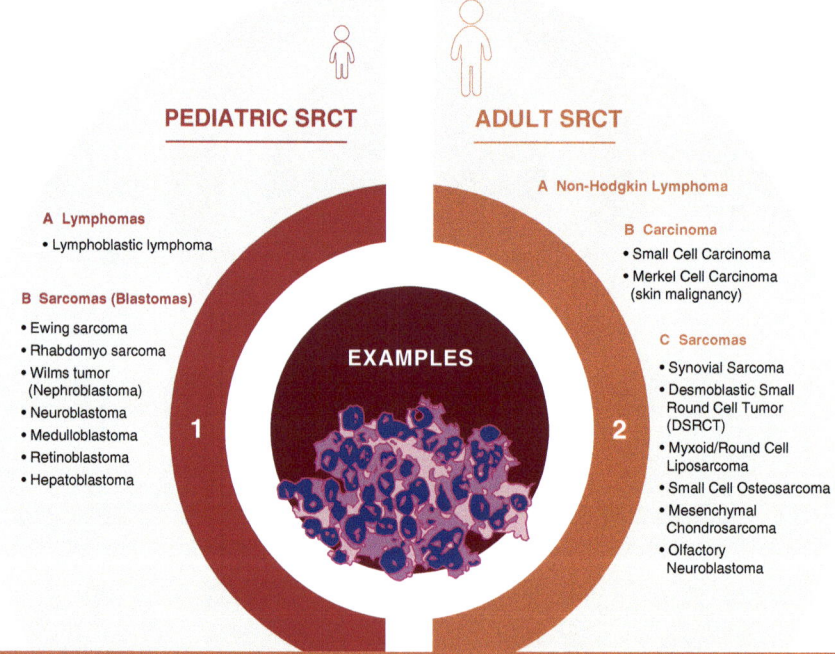

EXAMPLES

1   2

SPINDLE CELL TUMORS

DEFINITIONS

A tumor composed of elongated cells with fusiform nuclei. The most common pattern in soft tissue (mesenchymal) neoplasms.

CONSIDERATIONS

First think soft tissue tumors, whether benign or malignant (sarcoma). However, there are spindle-cell variants of both carcinomas & melanomas (uncommon variants).

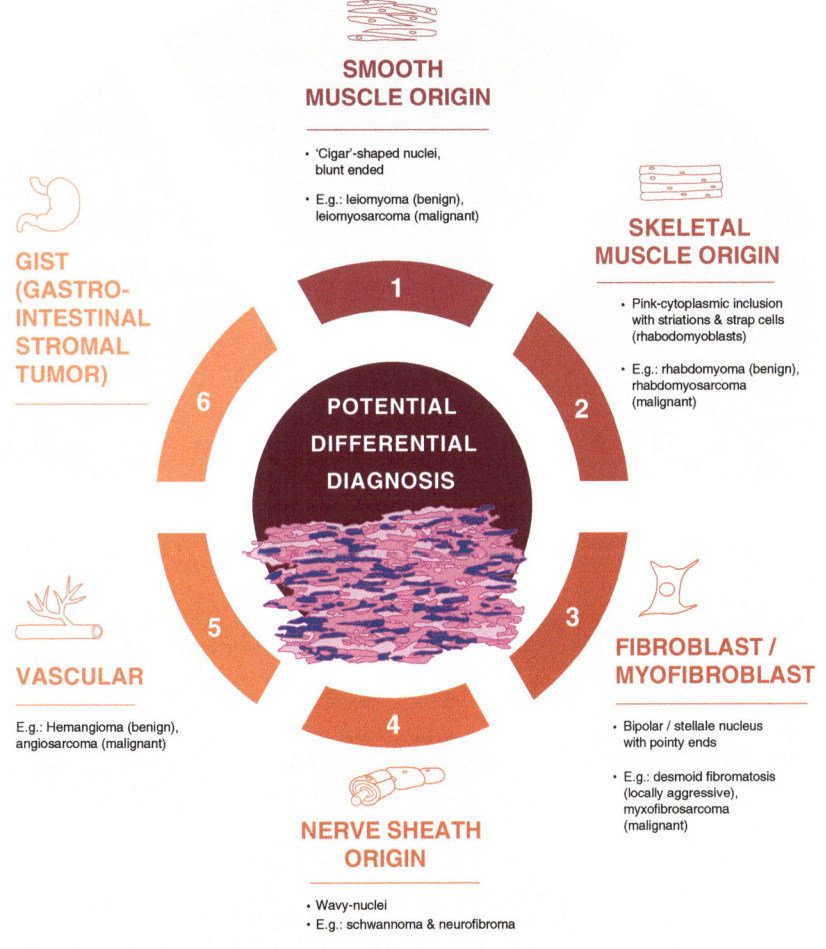

SMOOTH MUSCLE ORIGIN

- 'Cigar'-shaped nuclei, blunt ended
- E.g.: leiomyoma (benign), leiomyosarcoma (malignant)

SKELETAL MUSCLE ORIGIN

- Pink-cytoplasmic inclusion with striations & strap cells (rhabdomyoblasts)
- E.g.: rhabdomyoma (benign), rhabdomyosarcoma (malignant)

GIST (GASTRO-INTESTINAL STROMAL TUMOR)

POTENTIAL DIFFERENTIAL DIAGNOSIS

FIBROBLAST / MYOFIBROBLAST

- Bipolar / stellate nucleus with pointy ends
- E.g.: desmoid fibromatosis (locally aggressive), myxofibrosarcoma (malignant)

VASCULAR

E.g.: Hemangioma (benign), angiosarcoma (malignant)

NERVE SHEATH ORIGIN

- Wavy-nuclei
- E.g.: schwannoma & neurofibroma

(b)Terminology used to describe architectural patterns

Table 5.1 Describing key-features of the architectural patterns and their corresponding prototypic neoplasms

Architectural pattern	Brief description	Prototypic neoplasm
Cribriform	Sieve-like regular spaces	Adenoid cystic carcinoma of salivary glands Breast cribriform ductal carcinoma in situ (DCSI)
Alveolar	Nests of cells with empty spaces resembling lung alveoli	Alveolar soft part sarcoma
Basaloid	Blue, tightly packed cells, resembling basal cell carcinoma	Basaloid squamous cell carcinoma Basal cell carcinoma
Fascicular	Streaming bundle of spindle cells that may intersect perpendicularly	Leiomyoma
Herringbone	Spindle cells fascicles intersecting at acute angles	Fibrosarcoma
Hobnailed cells	Cells projecting into vascular lumina resembling a large-headed nail	Angiosarcoma
Microcystic pattern	Small cystic spaces	Serous cystadenoma of the pancreas Acinic cell carcinoma of salivary glands
Papillary	Finger-like projections containing fibrovascular cores	Papillary thyroid carcinoma
Micropapillary	Papillary-shaped small Epithelial projections without fibrovascular cores	Serous carcinoma of the ovary
Rosette	Radial arrangement of cells around a central point	Neuroblastic, neuroendocrine, or ependymal tumors Others: rosette-like structure can be seen in ovarian granulosa cell tumor (Call–Exner bodies)
Staghorn	Thin-walled branched vessels that have antler-like/staghorn shape	Solitary fibrous tumor
Storiform	Spindle cells Radiating outward from a central point (cartwheel pattern)	Dermatofibrosarcoma Protuberans (DFSP)

CRIBRIFORM

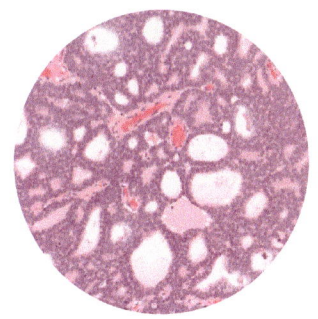 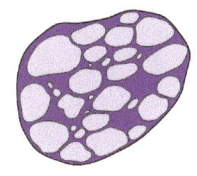 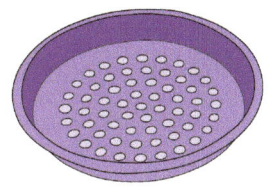

ALVEOLAR

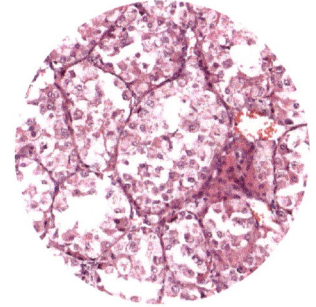 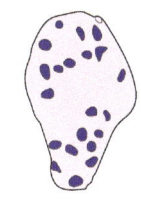 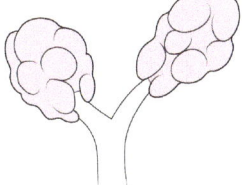

BASALOID

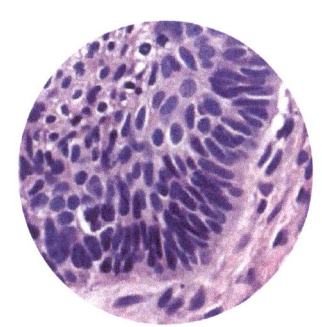 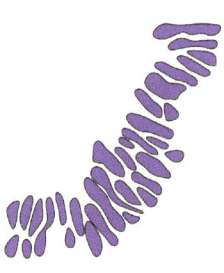 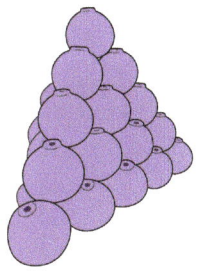

FASCICULAR PATTERN

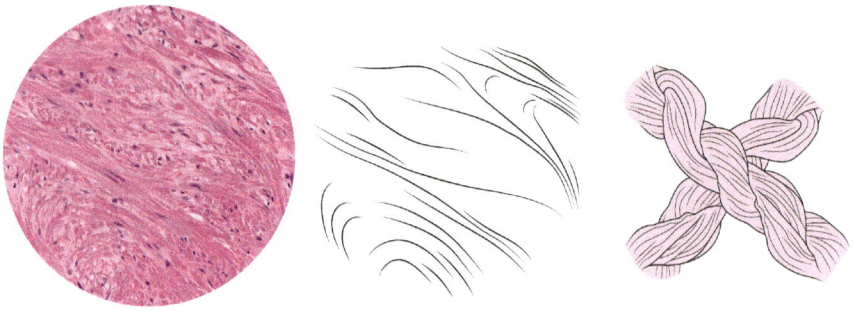

HERRINGBONE PATTERN

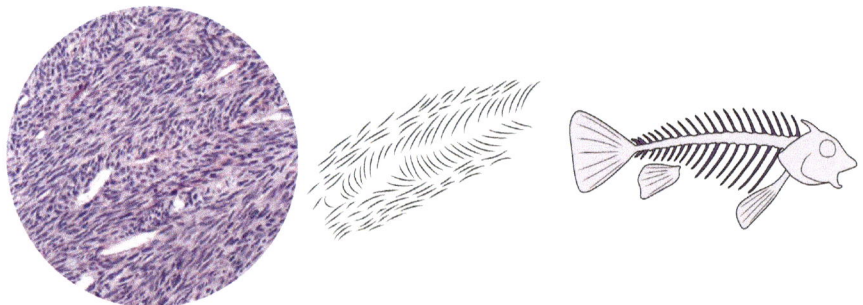

HOBNAILED CELLS

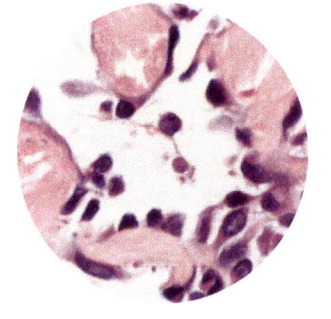 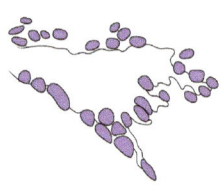 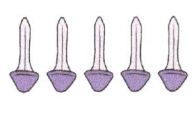

MICROCYSTIC PATTERN

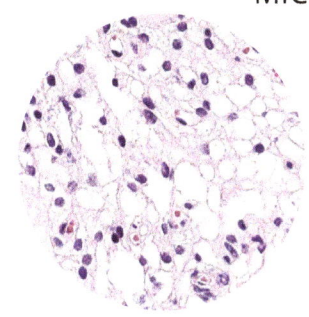 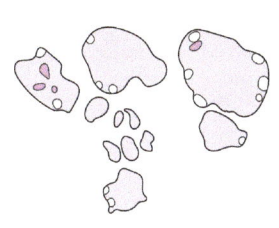 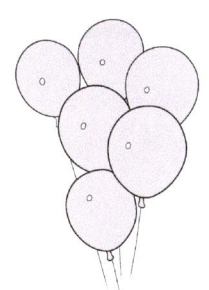

PAPILLARY ARCHITECTURE

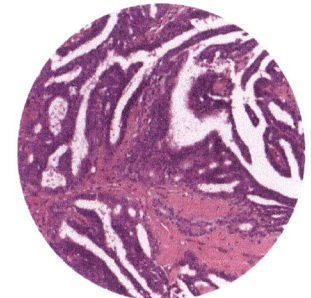 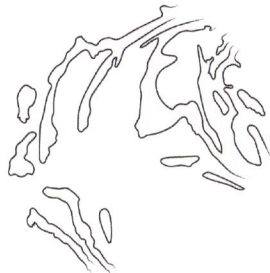 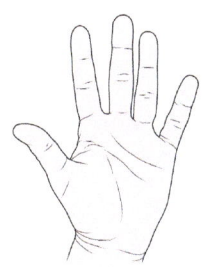

MICROPAPILLARY ARCHITECTURE

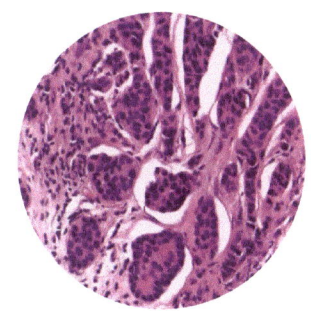 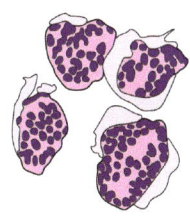 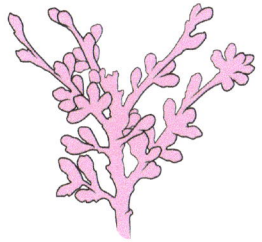

ROSETTE

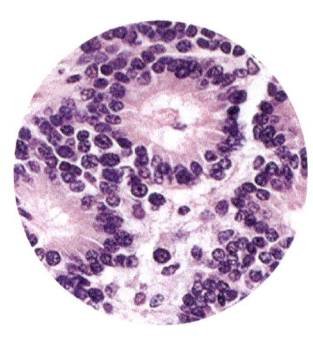 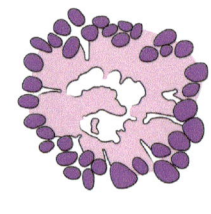 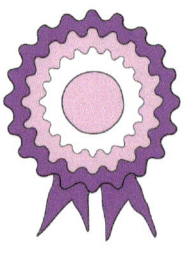

STAGHORN VESSELS

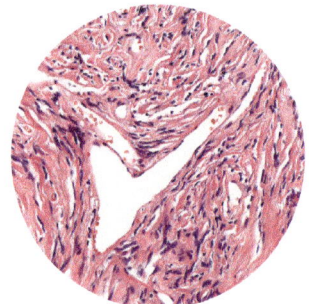 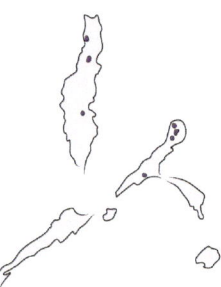 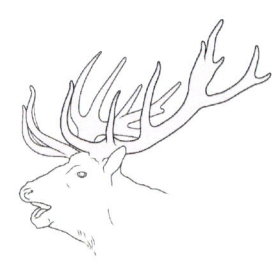

STORIFORM PATTERN

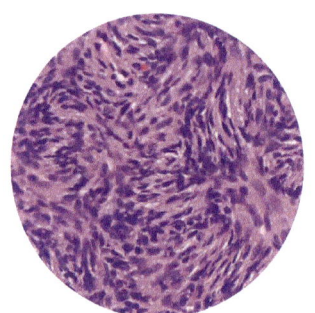 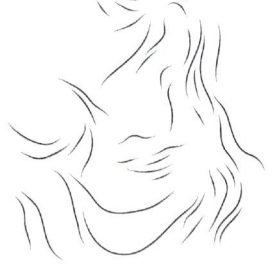 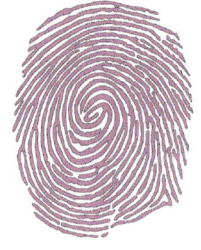

(c) Terminology used to describe pathologic processes

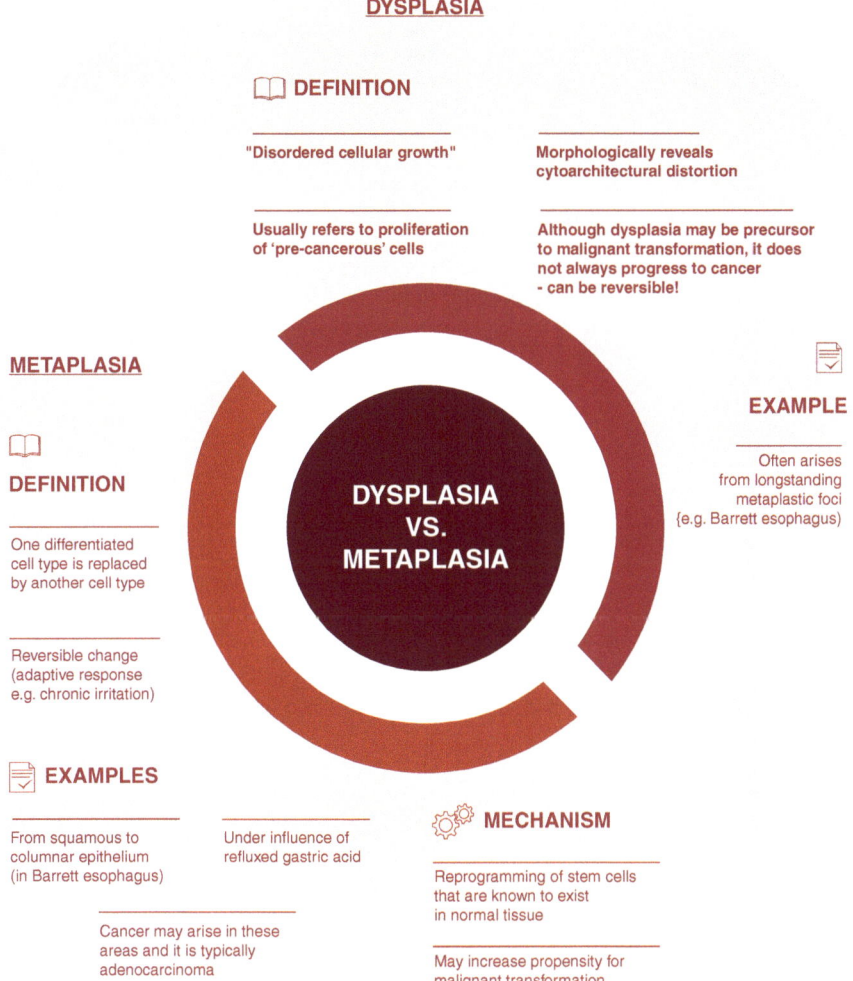

DYSPLASIA & METAPLASIA

DYSPLASIA

📖 **DEFINITION**

"Disordered cellular growth"

Morphologically reveals cytoarchitectural distortion

Usually refers to proliferation of 'pre-cancerous' cells

Although dysplasia may be precursor to malignant transformation, it does not always progress to cancer - can be reversible!

METAPLASIA

📖 **DEFINITION**

One differentiated cell type is replaced by another cell type

Reversible change (adaptive response e.g. chronic irritation)

📋 **EXAMPLES**

From squamous to columnar epithelium (in Barrett esophagus)

Under influence of refluxed gastric acid

Cancer may arise in these areas and it is typically adenocarcinoma

⚙ **MECHANISM**

Reprogramming of stem cells that are known to exist in normal tissue

May increase propensity for malignant transformation

DYSPLASIA VS. METAPLASIA

📋 **EXAMPLE**

Often arises from longstanding metaplastic foci (e.g. Barrett esophagus)

GRANULOMA & GRANULATION TISSUE

GRANULOMA

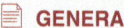 **GENERAL** → Granulomatous inflammation: a form of chronic inflammation

DEFINITION → collection of activated macrophages ± T-lymphocytes

WHY DOES IT FORM? → Attempt to contain an offending agent (that is difficult to eradicate)

*Some activated macrophages fuse → multinucleated giant cells

 TYPES

Foreian body garanuloma
form around (inert)
material e.g. suture

Immune granuloma
Inciting agent: persistent
microbe or self antigen

EXAMPLES

Infectious disease
• Tuberculosis:
Necrotizing (caseating)
granuloma ZN Stain:
Acid fast bacilli
• Leprosy
• Cat-scratch disease
Non-Infectious
• Sarcoidosis
• Crohn disease
• Foreign body
granuloma

GRANULATION TISSUE

DEFINITION

Proliferation of
fibroblasts+ capillaries
(angiogenesis)
in a loose matrix
± Inlammatory cells

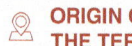 **ORIGIN OF THE TERM**

Grossly, it looks pink,
soft and granular (seen beneath
the scab of a skin wound)

GRANULOMA VS. GRANULATION TISSUE

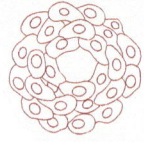

WHY DOES IT FORM?

Tissue repair process → invades the site of injury
Larger wound/defect requires a greater volume of granulation tissue to
fill in gaps → provide the underlying framework for regrowth of epithelium

HYPERPLASIA & HYPERTROPHY

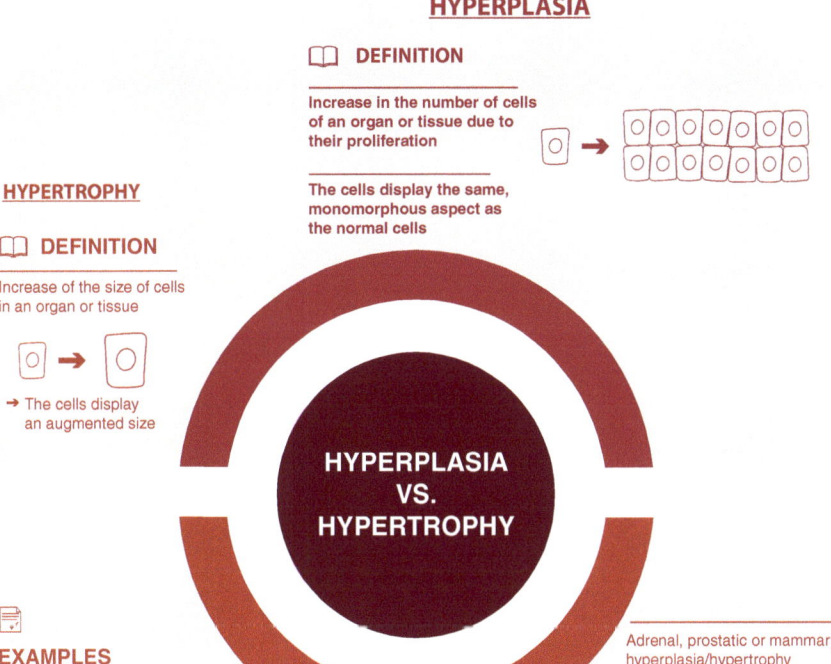

HYPERPLASIA

📖 **DEFINITION**

Increase in the number of cells
of an organ or tissue due to
their proliferation

The cells display the same,
monomorphous aspect as
the normal cells

HYPERTROPHY

📖 **DEFINITION**

Increase of the size of cells
in an organ or tissue

➔ The cells display
an augmented size

**HYPERPLASIA
VS.
HYPERTROPHY**

📑 **EXAMPLES**

Both are different adaption mechanisms
of cells against stress(mechanic, hormonal...),
occur often simultaneously and result
in the enlargement of the organ or tissue

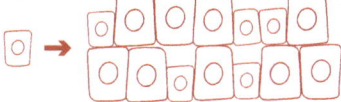

Adrenal, prostatic or mammary
hyperplasia/hypertrophy

In some organs, the term hyperplasia may
have a somewhat blurry distinction from benign
neoplastic lesions (e.g: adenoma) because both
conditions results from a cellular proliferation, which,
however, might be mono- or polyclonal. Most of the
time hyperplasia refers to the diffuse enlargement of
an organ (ex.: goiter) while adenoma refers to a more
delimited nodule within an organ (ex.: thyroid adenoma)

Sometimes, the hyperplasia can display cellular atypia,
which is related to a higher occurrence of neoplasia
or is a precursor lesion of cancer (e.g.: uterine
atypical endometrial hyperplasia
→ endometrioid endometrial
carcinoma)

Further Reading

Abbas AK, Aster JC, Kumar V. Robbins and Cotran pathologic basis of disease. Philadelphia: Elsevier/Saunders; 2015.

Molavi DW. The practice of surgical pathology: a beginners guide to the diagnostic process. Cham: Springer International Publishing; 2018.

Rekhtman N, Bishop JA. Quick reference handbook for surgical pathologists. Berlin: Springer; 2011.

Rubin E, Reisner HM. Essentials of Rubin's pathology. Philadelphia: Lippincott Williams & Wilkins; 2013.

Part III

The Journey of Specimens

The Journey of Specimens: From the Operating Table to the Microscope

6

Ahmad Altaleb

Objective

- Understand the "big picture" of the basic steps carried out at the pathology laboratory in order to obtain glass slides, by illustrating the specimen's route all the way from the operation room to the pathologist's microscope.

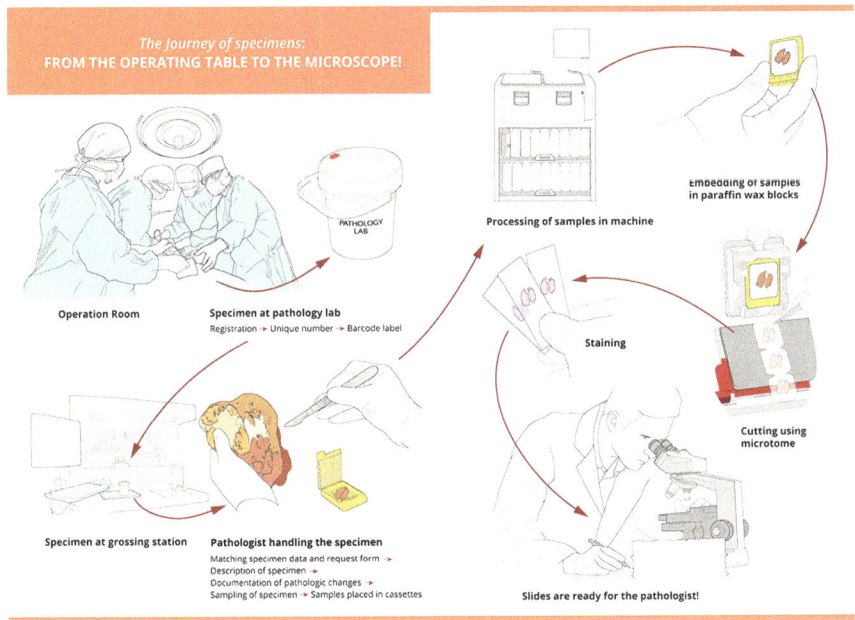

The Journey of specimens:
FROM THE OPERATING TABLE TO THE MICROSCOPE!

Operation Room

Specimen at pathology lab
Registration → Unique number → Barcode label

Processing of samples in machine

Embedding of samples in paraffin wax blocks

Cutting using microtome

Staining

Specimen at grossing station

Pathologist handling the specimen
Matching specimen data and request form →
Description of specimen →
Documentation of pathologic changes →
Sampling of specimen → Samples placed in cassettes

Slides are ready for the pathologist!

A. Altaleb (✉)
Histopathology Department, Mubarak Alkabeer Hospital, Jabriya, Kuwait

A. Altaleb (ed.), *Surgical Pathology*,
https://doi.org/10.1007/978-3-030-53690-9_6

At the Grossing Station: Principles of Specimen Handling and Cut-Up

Ahmad Altaleb

Objective

- Learn the setup of the grossing area and how the pathologist handles the specimens at the grossing area

A. Altaleb (✉)
Histopathology Department, Mubarak Alkabeer Hospital, Jabriya, Kuwait

AT THE GROSSING STATION

After specimen registration and obtaining a unique ID number it arrives at the grossing area (for gross examination and sampling). The pathologist ensures that the info on the request form matches the info on the specimen container.

THE PATHOLOGIST...

(1) orients the specimen by identifying anatomic structures or surgical sutures inserted by the surgeon

(2) measures the specimen (some specimens should take weight too).

(3) inks the margins (most large specimens).

(4) dissects the specimen by serial sectioning (solid organs) or opening (bowel) for identifying the pathologic process.

(5) describes the pathologic process (size, color, consistency, shape, distance form margin(s)), status of margins, and other relevant findings.

(6) takes samples (from the lesion, margins and relevant non–lesional areas) for microscope examination.

GENERAL NOTES

· Adequate formalin fixation (usually 24 hours or overnight) is mandatory for all specimens.
· Biopsy specimens need less time: ~ 6 – 8 hours.

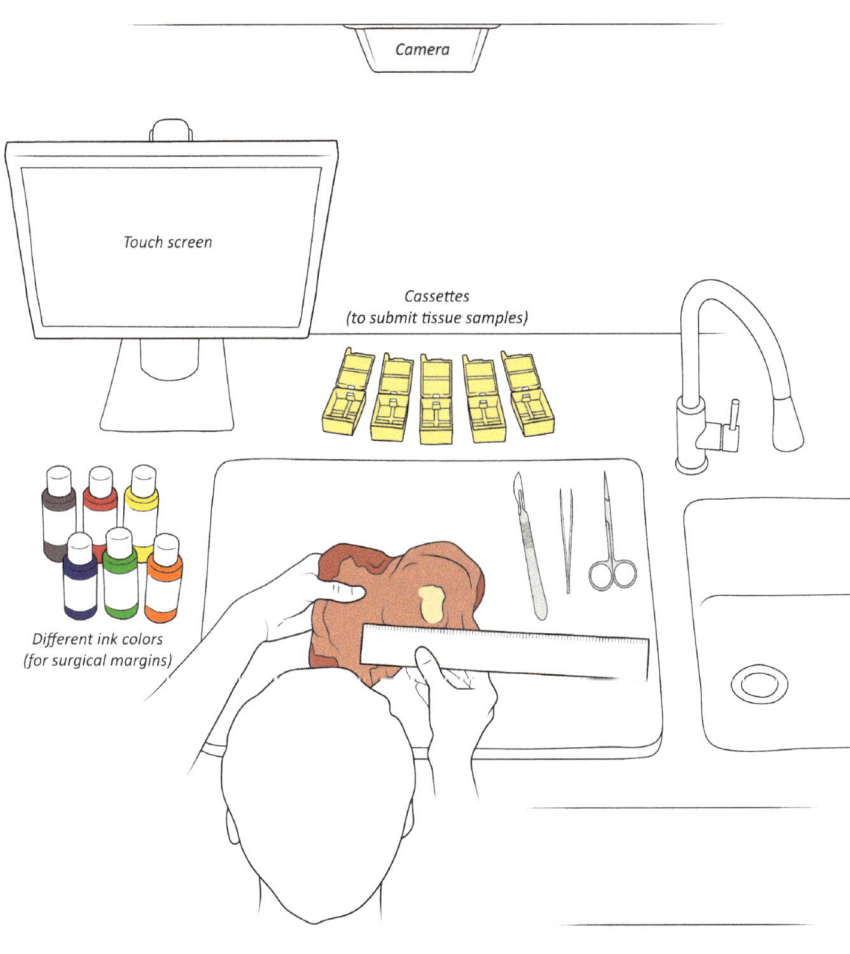

Fig. 7.1 The overall setting of the grossing area. The illustration depicts the pathologist describing the gross/macroscopic findings

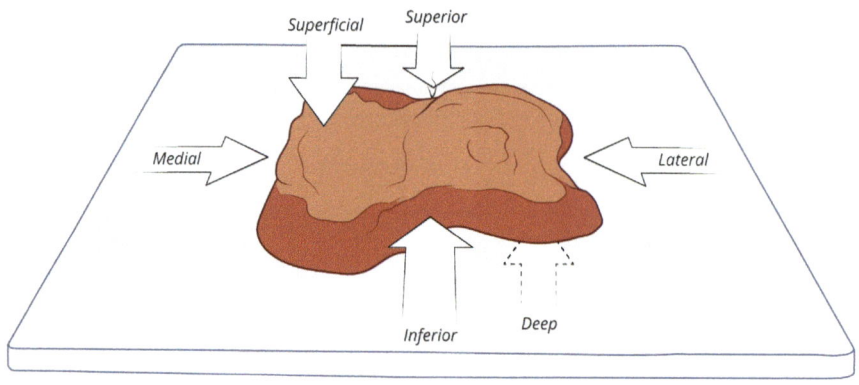

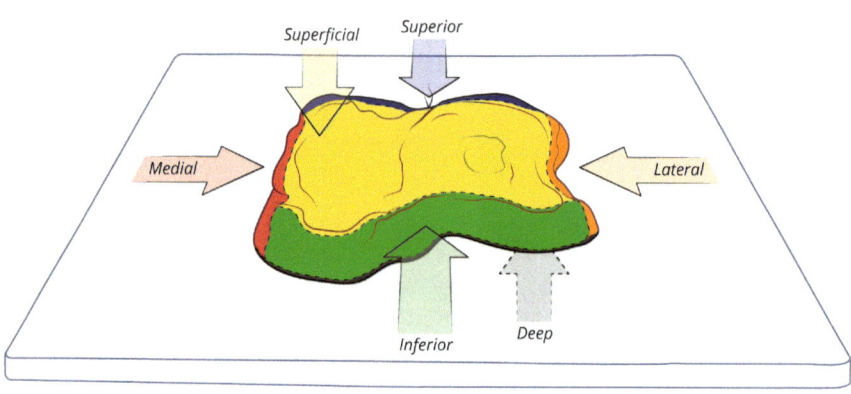

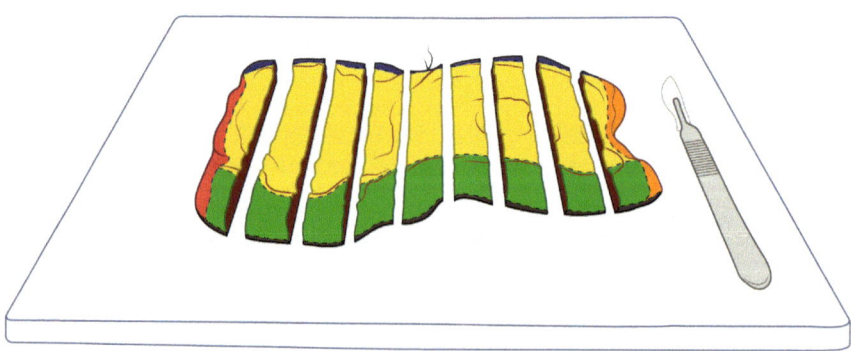

Fig. 7.2 Basic steps of specimen orientation, by differential inking, for surgical margin assessment of a lumpectomy specimen (e.g., *wide local excision (WLE)* of breast carcinoma). Specimen orientation **(top)**. Surgical sutures are usually inserted at different aspects of the specimen to guide the pathologist orienting the specimen correctly; a diagram attached to the request form may aid this. Specimen inking **(middle)**. Different colors are recommended to ink each margin to assess the adequacy of the excision. Serial sectioning **(bottom)**—a step just before sampling of the specimen/lesion

Basics of Tissue Processing

Ahmad Altaleb

Objective

- Learn about the steps of tissue processing and obtaining glass slides.

A. Altaleb (✉)
Histopathology Department, Mubarak Alkabeer Hospital, Jabriya, Kuwait

TISSUE PROCESSING

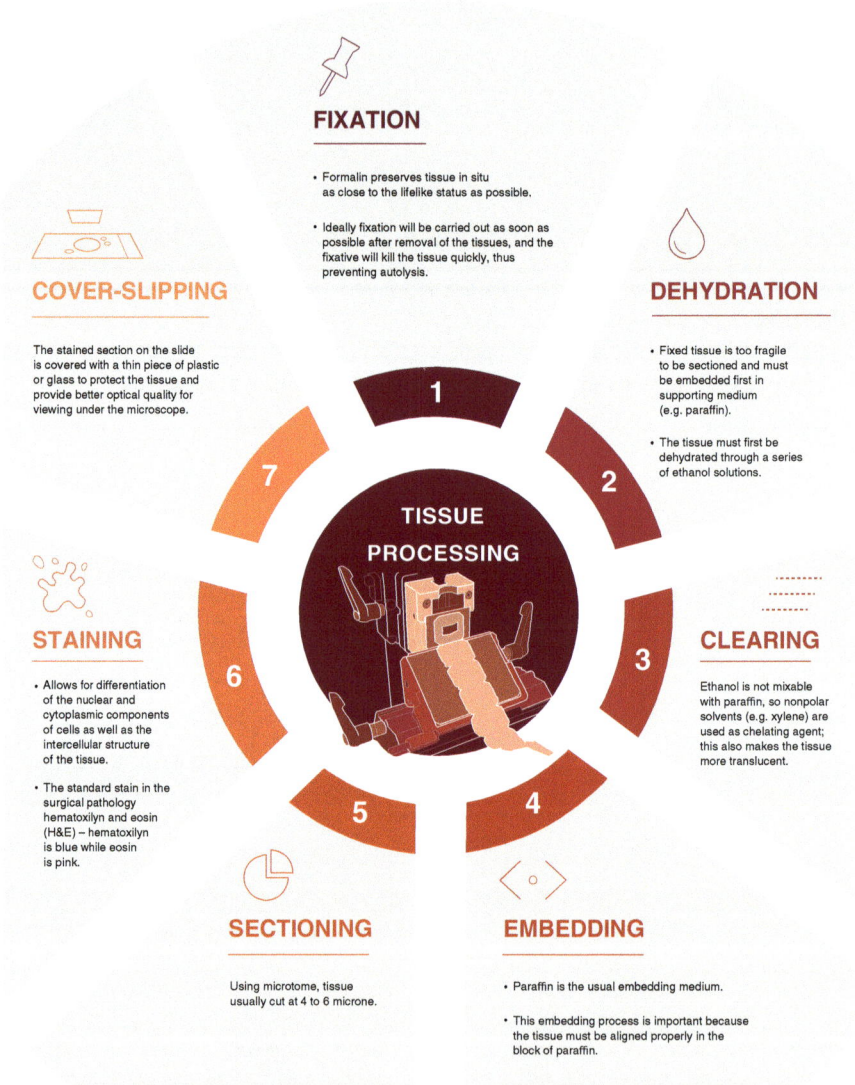

FIXATION

- Formalin preserves tissue in situ as close to the lifelike status as possible.

- Ideally fixation will be carried out as soon as possible after removal of the tissues, and the fixative will kill the tissue quickly, thus preventing autolysis.

COVER-SLIPPING

The stained section on the slide is covered with a thin piece of plastic or glass to protect the tissue and provide better optical quality for viewing under the microscope.

DEHYDRATION

- Fixed tissue is too fragile to be sectioned and must be embedded first in supporting medium (e.g. paraffin).

- The tissue must first be dehydrated through a series of ethanol solutions.

STAINING

- Allows for differentiation of the nuclear and cytoplasmic components of cells as well as the intercellular structure of the tissue.

- The standard stain in the surgical pathology hematoxilyn and eosin (H&E) – hematoxilyn is blue while eosin is pink.

CLEARING

Ethanol is not mixable with paraffin, so nonpolar solvents (e.g. xylene) are used as chelating agent; this also makes the tissue more translucent.

SECTIONING

Using microtome, tissue usually cut at 4 to 6 microne.

EMBEDDING

- Paraffin is the usual embedding medium.

- This embedding process is important because the tissue must be aligned properly in the block of paraffin.

TISSUE PROCESSING

1 2 3 4 5 6 7

Further Reading

Gattuso P. Differential diagnosis in surgical pathology. Philadelphia: Saunders/Elsevier; 2015.

Lester SC. Manual of surgical pathology: expert consult. 3rd ed. Philadelphia: Elsevier/ Saunders; 2010.

A Primer on Gross Pathology Examination and Selected Images of Gross Specimens

Ahmad Altaleb

Objective

- Learn about basic methods the pathologist uses to analyze surgical specimens and identify the macroscopic changes.
- Study some gross/macroscopic features of selected surgical pathology specimens

Specimens received from the operation room are usually the first encounter (and probably the last!) between the pathologist and the patient. They might be sent either fixed (e.g., in formalin) or unfixed (fresh). In either case, the pathologist has to handle the surgical specimens very carefully. This is because a good gross description and sampling is a prerequisite for an accurate final diagnosis.

In many instances, the use of photographs or diagrams for mapping the specimens would be of great help to ascertain the pathologic process and assess its extent (e.g., breast lumpectomies for ductal carcinoma in situ).

After orienting the specimen, it should be placed on a cutting board in anatomic position and record certain points like the type of the specimen, structures included, dimensions, and identify any pathologic process present before dissection. Then the pathologist has to open the specimen and identify the lesion or pathologic process present and describe it (see Chap. 7).

The pathologist primarily relies on inspection skills as well as palpation to identify and elucidate the pathologic processes present in the surgical specimen.

Usually, there are clues present in the specimen to identify the gross pathologic alterations. These could be a change in the *shape, color, consistency,* or even the *size* of an organ or tissue (Figs. 9.1, 9.2, and 9.3). It is often the *constellation* of these

A. Altaleb (✉)
Histopathology Department, Mubarak Alkabeer Hospital, Jabriya, Kuwait

© The Editor(s) (if applicable) and The Author(s), under exclusive license to Springer Nature Switzerland AG 2021
A. Altaleb (ed.), *Surgical Pathology*,
https://doi.org/10.1007/978-3-030-53690-9_9

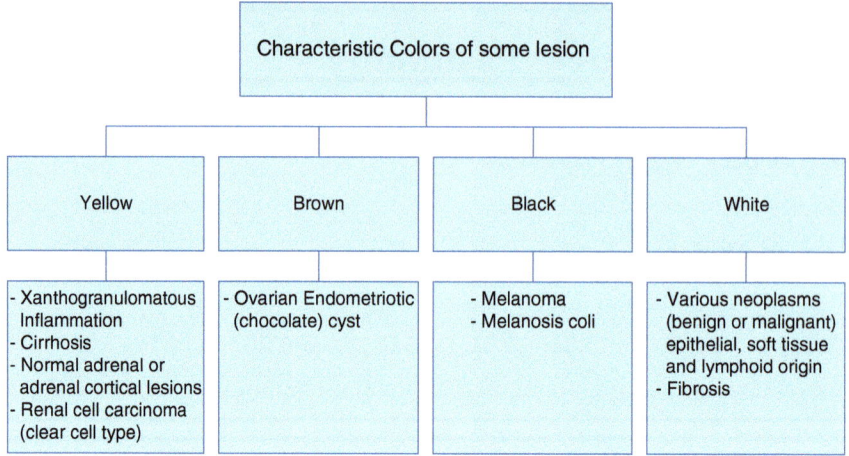

Fig. 9.1 Characteristic colors of some lesion seen on gross examination

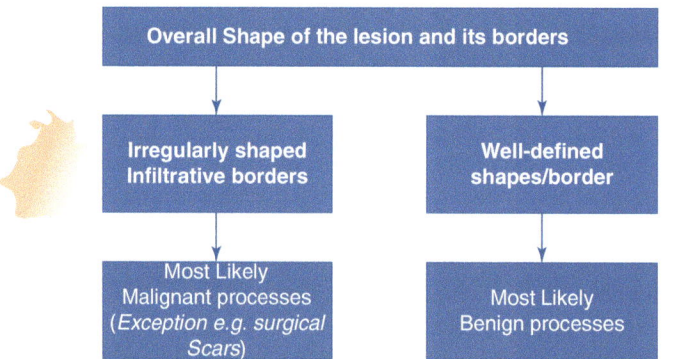

Fig. 9.2 Characteristic shape and border of lesion seen on gross examination

features that help to reach a macroscopic impression at the time of gross examination of surgical specimens. See gross images examples (Figs. 9.4, 9.5, 9.6, 9.7, 9.8, 9.9, 9.10, 9.11, 9.12, 9.13, 9.14, 9.15, 9.16, 9.17, 9.18, 9.19, 9.20, 9.21, 9.22, and 9.23).

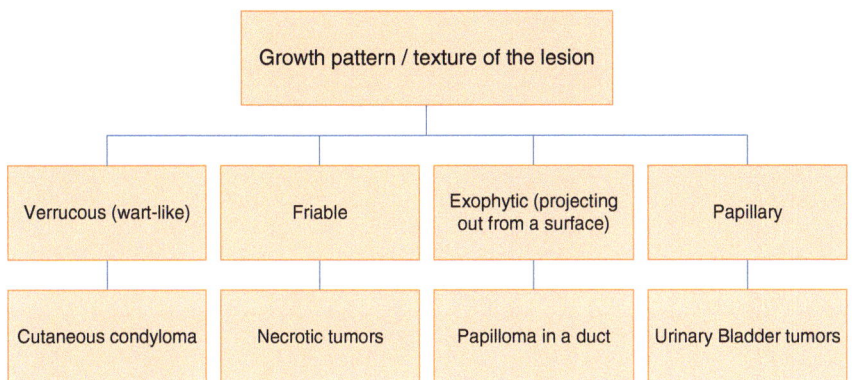

Fig. 9.3 Characteristic growth pattern/texture of lesions seen on gross examination

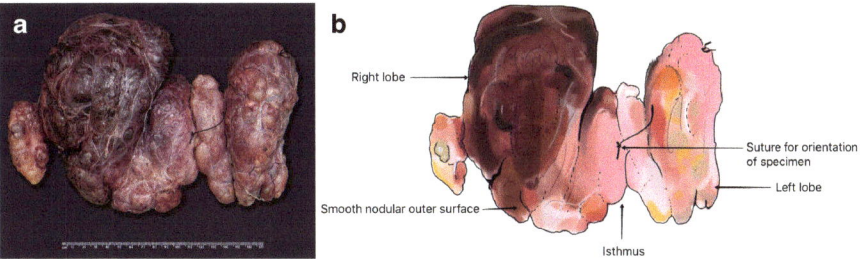

Fig. 9.4 Thyroidectomy specimen of a 50-year-old female with *nodular hyperplasia (multinodular goiter)*. (**a**) The gland is asymmetrically enlarged and distorted. Anterior view of the thyroid gland (0.5 kg). (**b**) Schematic diagram. (Illustrations are by lead author Dr. Ahmad Altaleb)

Fig. 9.5 A 23-year-old female presented with a painless, firm, mobile, slow-growing breast mass. Lumpectomy specimen: cut surface shows a well-circumscribed, white mass with lobulations bulge above the cut surface and occasional slit-like spaces. *Diagnosis: Fibroadenoma*

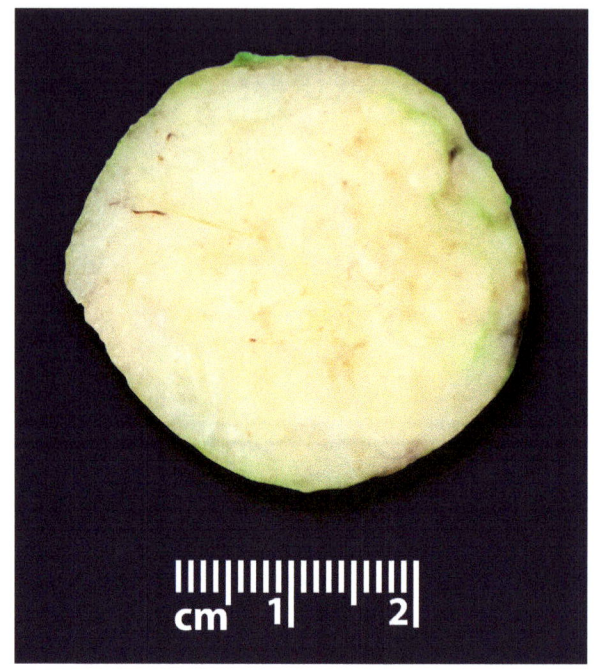

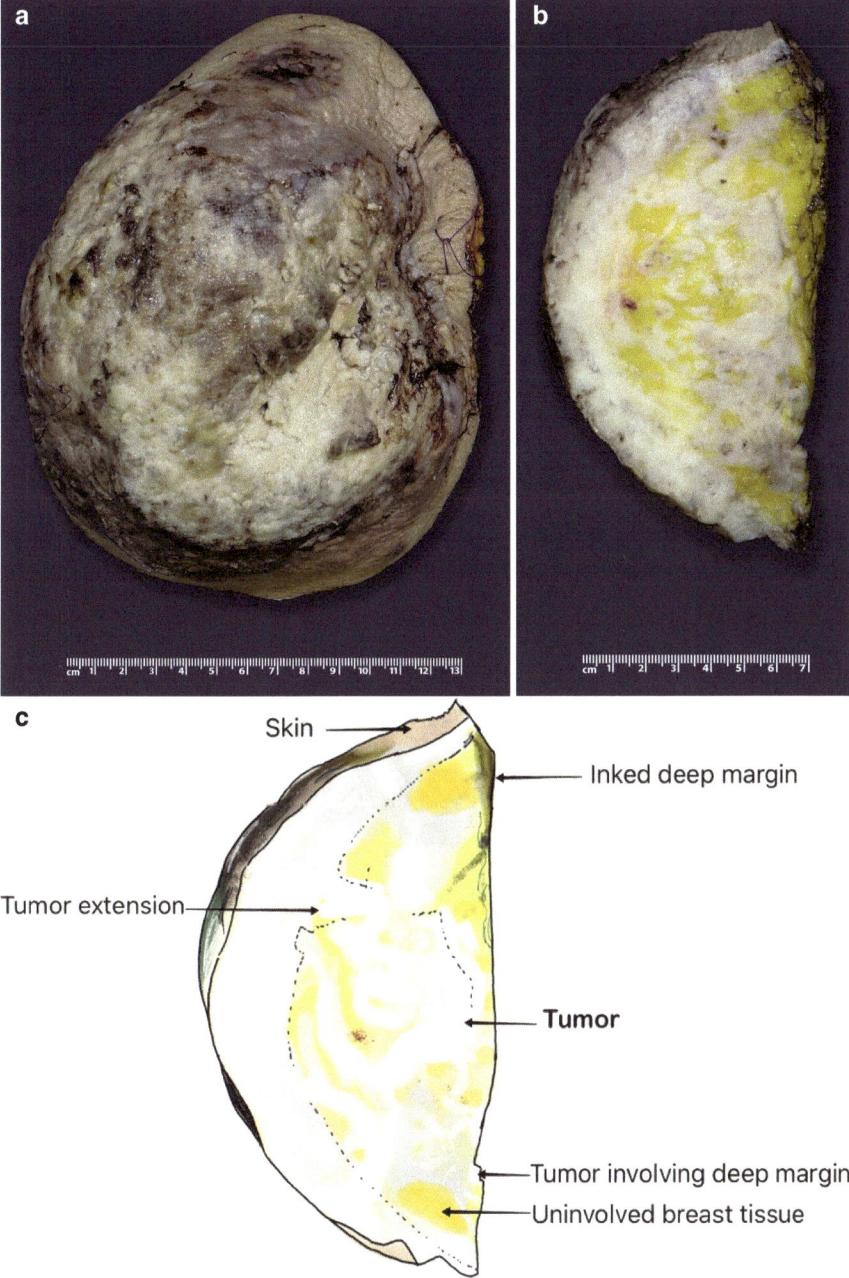

Fig. 9.6 A 61-year-old female presented with septicemia and found to have a locally advanced breast cancer. She underwent an "emergency life saving" mastectomy. (**a**) The skin of the breast is extensively involved by the tumor with areas of ulceration and necrosis. The nipple–areola complex couldn't be identified. (**b**) Cut section of the specimen shows a tumor almost involving the entire breast with cutaneous extension. Notice the positive deep surgical margin. (**c**) Schematic diagram. *Diagnosis: Invasive ductal carcinoma, grade 3, pT4b*

Fig. 9.7 A 14-year-old male with *Meckel's diverticulum.* Notice the anti-mesenteric 3.3 cm outpouching

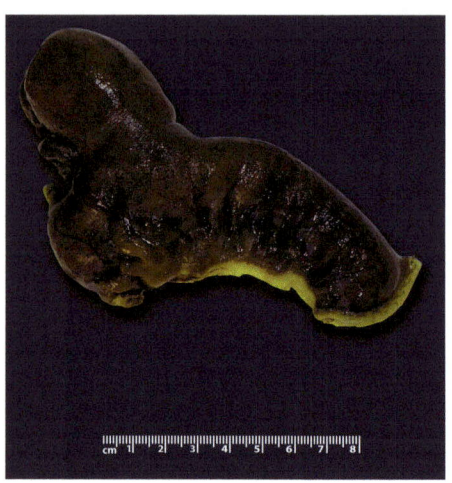

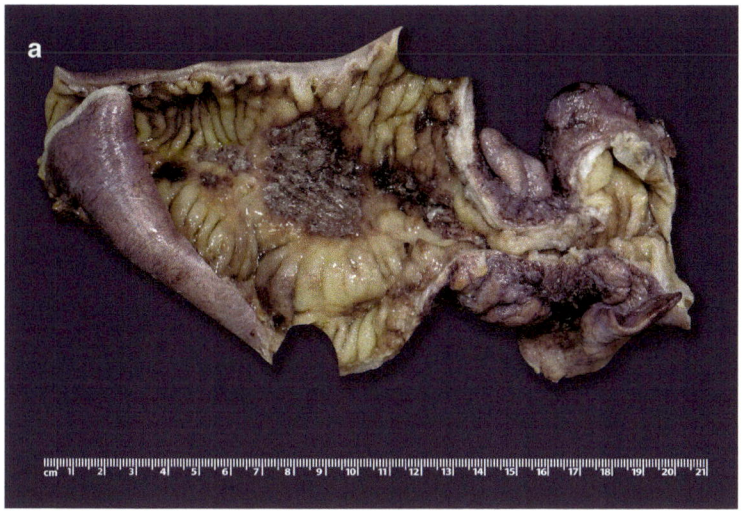

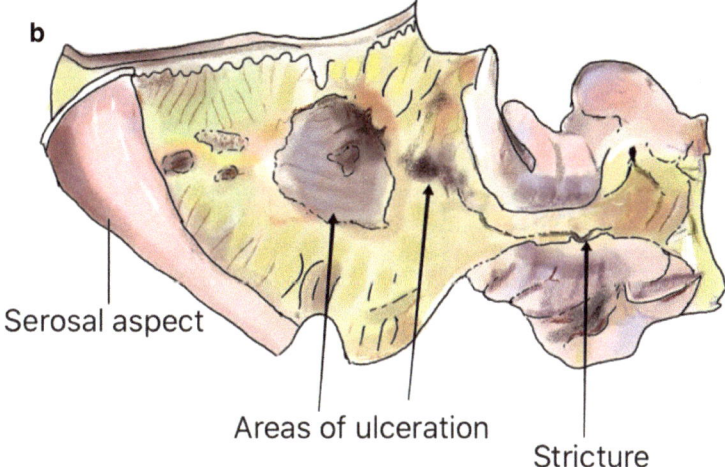

Fig. 9.8 A 22-year-old male known case of *Crohn disease* presented with bowel obstruction. (**a**) Limited right hemicolectomy, opened specimen; ileum with ulceration, and luminal stricture. (**b**) Schematic diagram

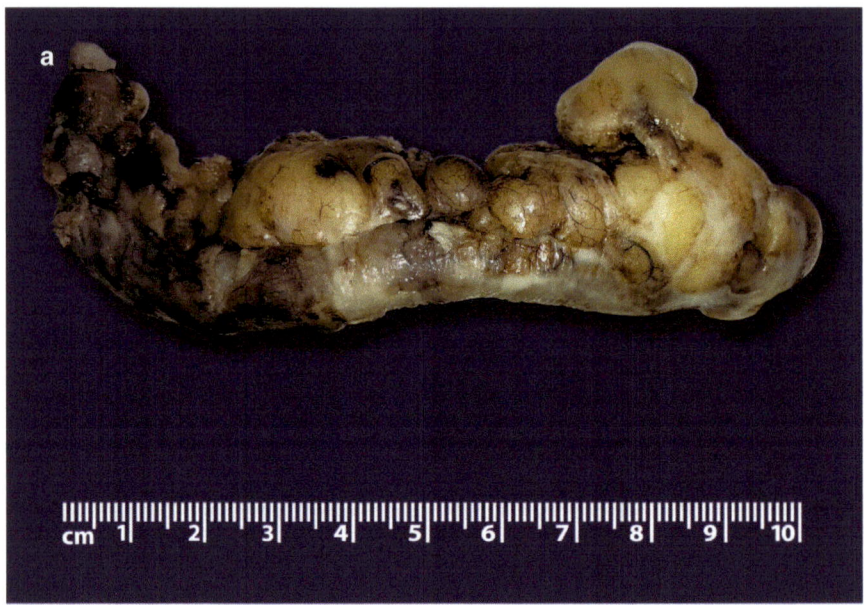

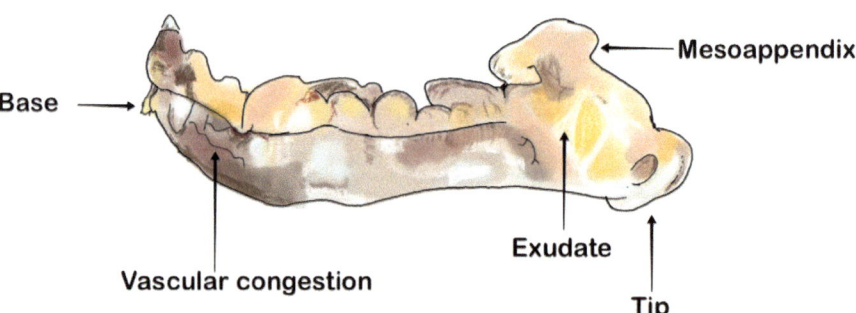

Fig. 9.9 A 19-year-old male presented with an acute abdomen underwent an appendectomy. (**a**) Notice the fibrinopurulent exudate on the surface and the focal serosal congestion. (**b**) Schematic diagram. *Diagnosis: Acute appendicitis*

Fig. 9.10 A 42-year-old female with recurrent biliary colic. Cholecystectomy specimen open longitudinally shows a rough mucosa with multiple yellow gallstones. *Diagnosis: Chronic cholecystitis with cholelithiasis*

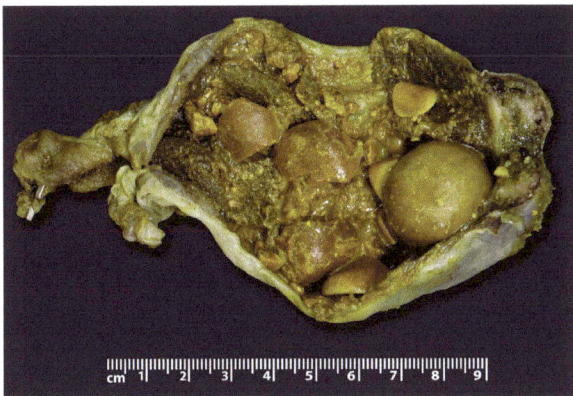

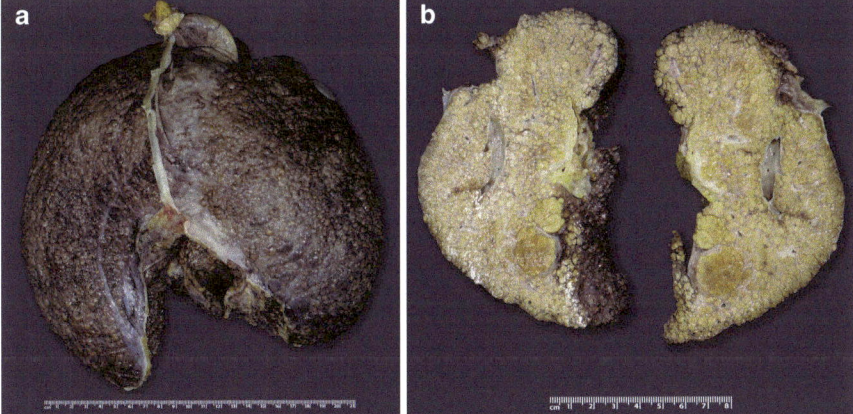

Fig. 9.11 A 42-year-old male with *liver cirrhosis* underwent liver transplantation. This is the explanted liver—measures 22 cm in maximum dimension and weighs 1.1 kg. Micronodular pattern of cirrhosis is evident. (**a**) External aspect, (**b**) Cut sections

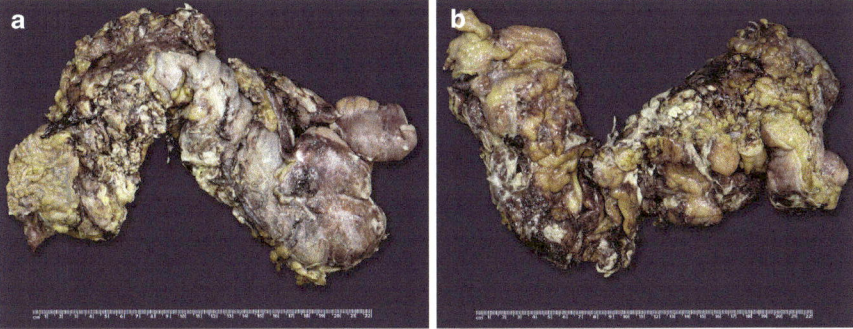

Fig. 9.12 A 67-year-old male underwent right hemicolectomy due to perforation? Etiology. The serosal surface shows extensive pale yellow fibrinopurulent exudate. The mucosa is unremarkable (not shown). A segment of the terminal ilium is present (specimen **a** upper right). (**a**) Anterior view. (**b**) Posterior view

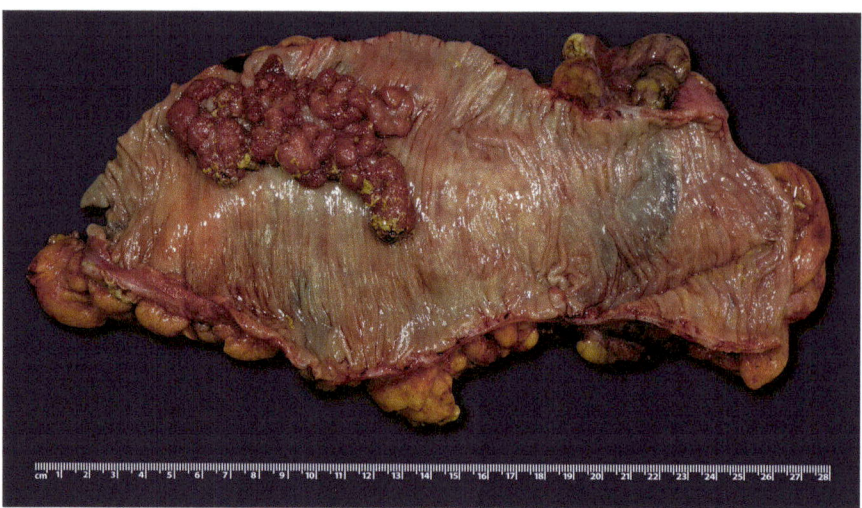

Fig. 9.13 A 63-year-old female underwent left hemicolectomy. This large polypoid mass (approx. 8.0 cm) represents a *tubulovillous adenoma with high-grade dysplasia*. No invasion is present after thorough sampling of the adenoma

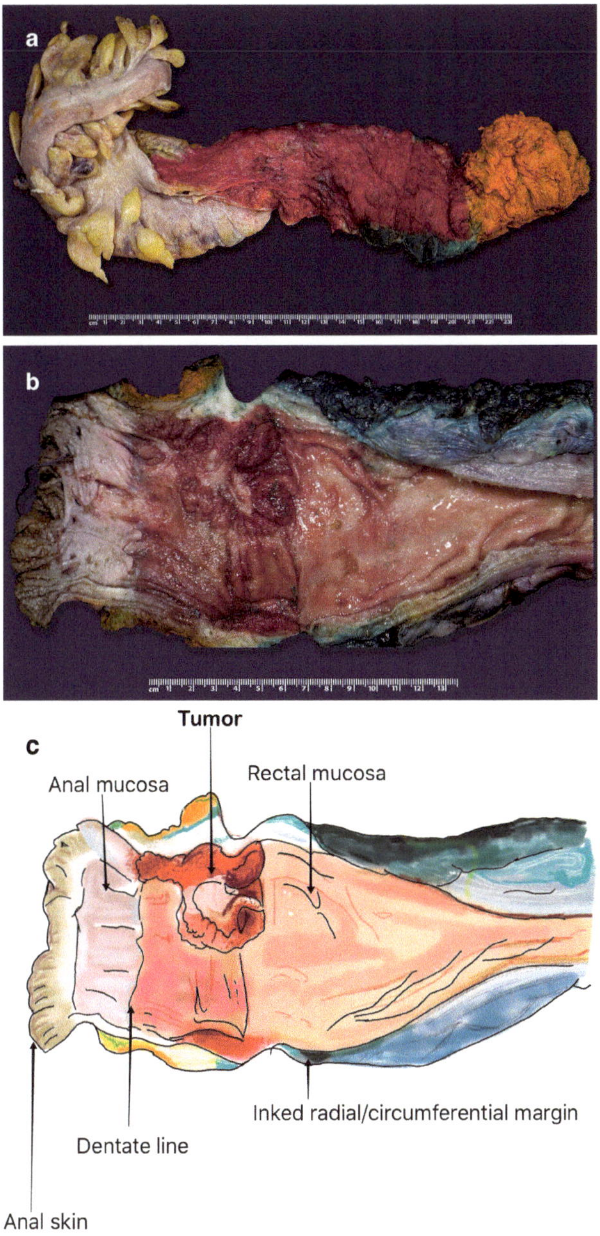

Fig. 9.14 A 77-year-old female with biopsy-proven low rectal cancer, status post neoadjuvant therapy. Abdominoperineal resection specimen. (**a**) Shows an ulcered rectal mass (3.0 cm in diameter). Microscopy shows a residual *well-differentiated adenocarcinoma* invading the submucosa, ypT1N0. Lymph nodes are negative for metastases. (**a**) Inked specimen before opening (postero-lateral view. Red: posterior mesorectum, green: anterior mesorectum). Inking is important for the evaluation of margins/adequacy of resection. In this example, the non-peritonealized bare area of the rectum represents the circumferential radial margin. (**b**) Opened specimen to show the mucosal/luminal aspect and the tumor. (**c**) Schematic diagram

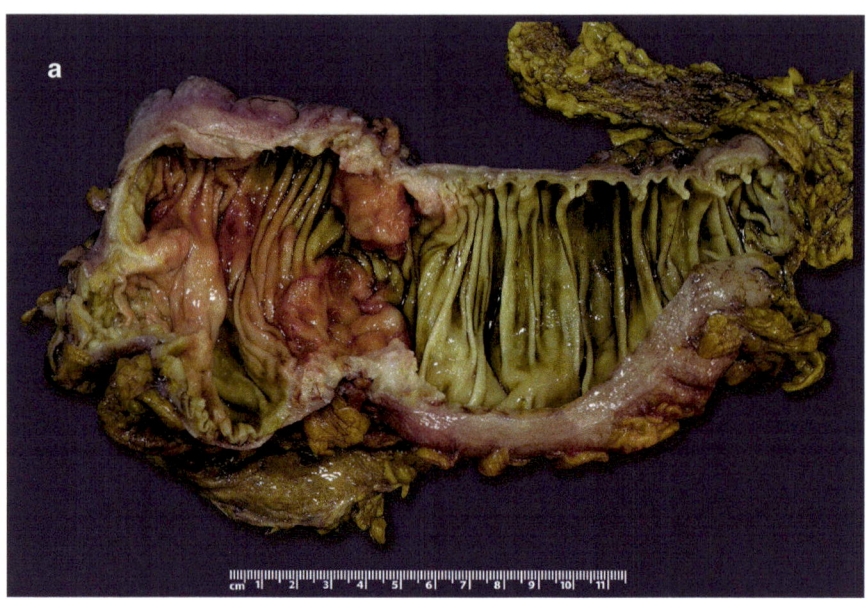

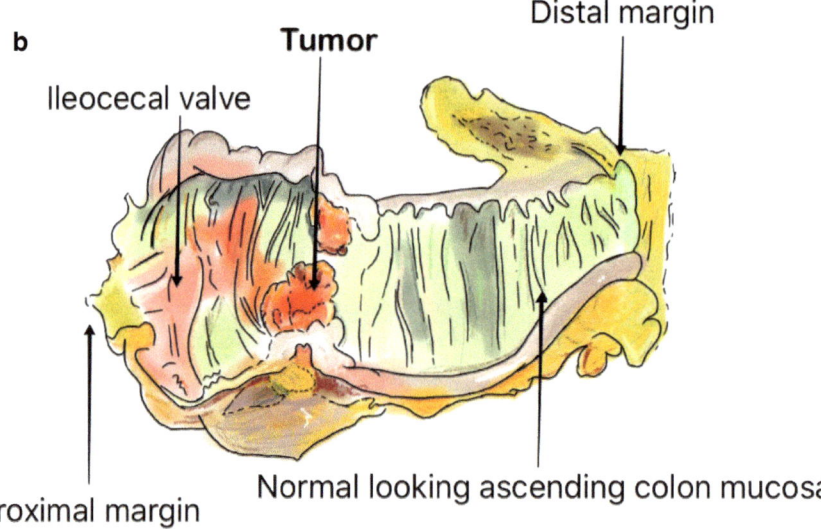

Fig. 9.15 A 69-year-old male with cecal mass underwent right hemicolectomy. There is a large fungating tumor (5 × 3 × 2 cm). Lymph nodes are negative for metastases. Diagnosis: *Adenocarcinoma pT4a N0*. (**a**) Opened specimen to show the mucosal/luminal aspect and the tumor. (**b**) Schematic diagram

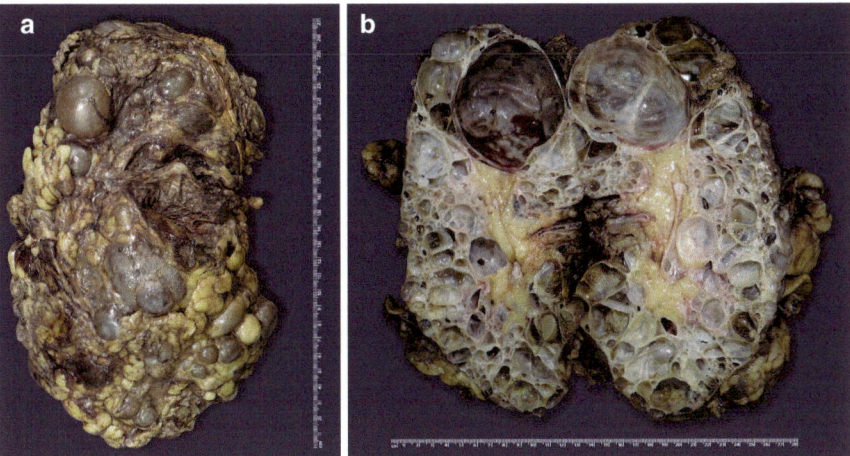

Fig. 9.16 Nephrectomy specimen of a 42-year-old male with end-stage renal disease secondary to *adult polycystic kidney disease*. Markedly enlarged kidney (weight = 2.4 kg and dimension = 27 cm). Outer aspect of the kidney shows bossolated surface. Cut surface shows numerous cysts replacing the renal parenchyma. (**a**) Outer aspect. (**b**) Cut surface of the kidney

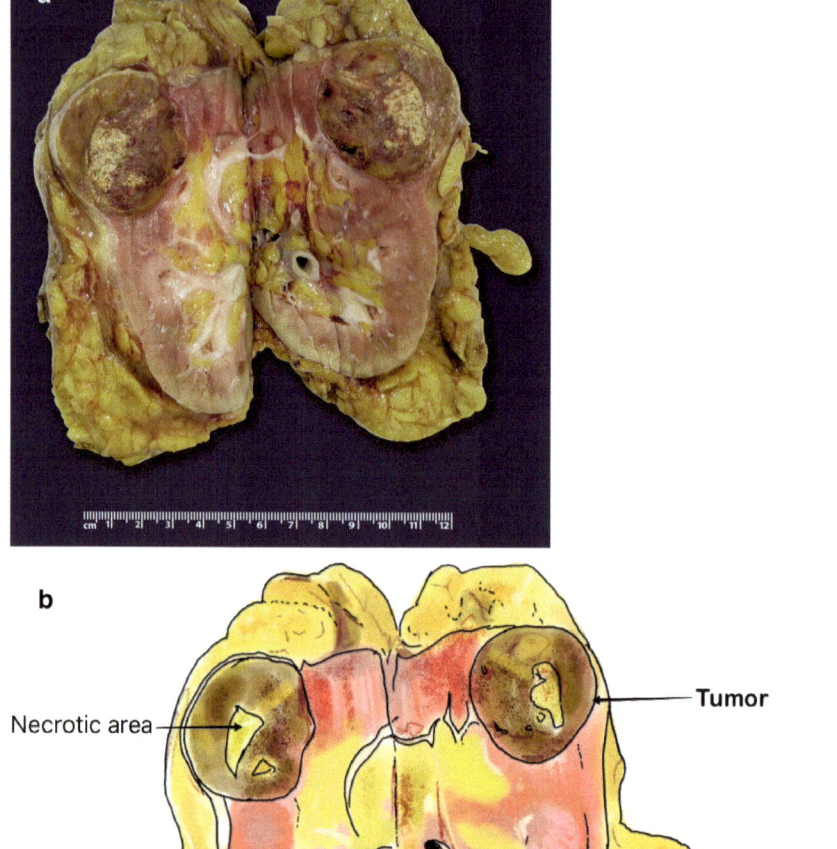

Fig. 9.17 A 75-year-old male with renal mass underwent nephrectomy. A 4 cm upper pole fleshy brown-red mass. *Diagnosis: Type 2 papillary renal cell carcinoma pT1a.* (**a**) A bivalved nephrectomy specimen shows the tumor at the upper pole. (**b**) Schematic diagram

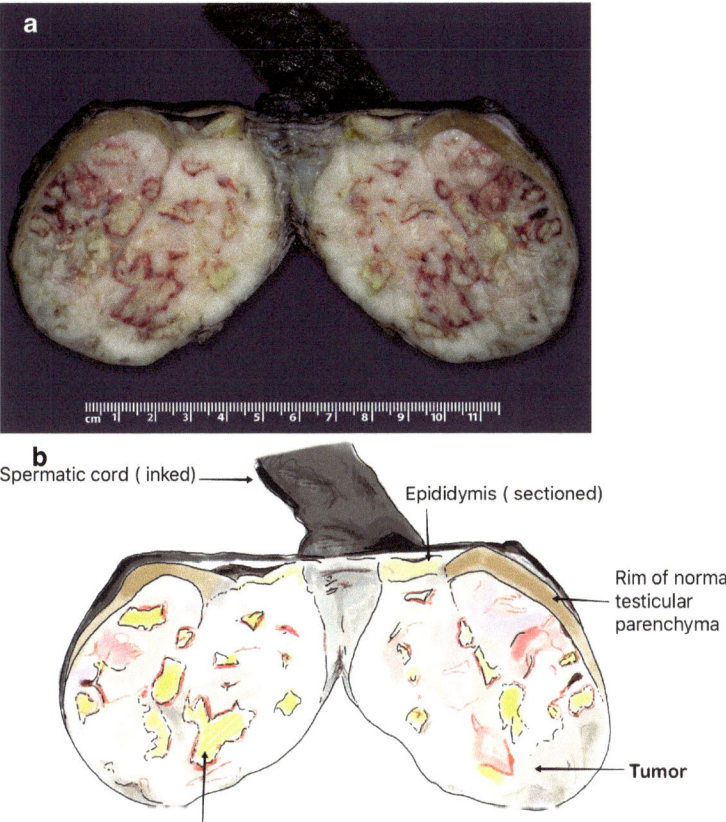

Spermatic cord (inked)

Epididymis (sectioned)

Rim of normal testicular parenchyma

Tumor

Islands of necrosis surrounded by hemorrhage

Fig. 9.18 Orchidectomy specimen of a 29-year-old male with a testicular tumor. The cut surface is variegated with yellow areas rimmed by thin hemorrhagic borders. Notice the uninvolved thin rim of testicular parenchyma at the periphery. Diagnosis: *Mixed germ cell tumor*, largely composed of seminoma with a minor component of embryonal carcinoma, pT1. (**a**) The cut surface of the testis. (**b**) Schematic diagram

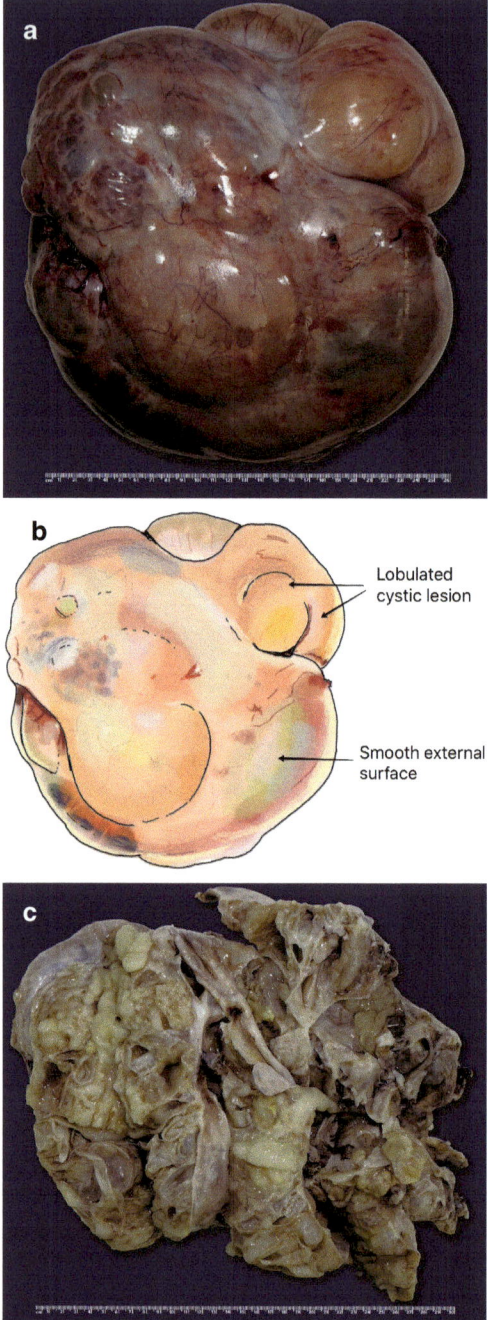

Fig. 9.19 A 35-year-old female presented with a pelviabdominal mass which appeared to be a large unilateral ovarian cystic lesion (29.0 cm in max. dimension). Diagnosis: *Ovarian mucinous carcinoma* pT1. (**a**) Outer surface. (**b**) Schematic diagram. (**c**) Inner aspect reveals a multilocular cyst containing thick mucinous material and solid areas

Fig. 9.20 A 46-year-old female with cervical lymphadenopathy (2.5 × 2.3 × 1.4 cm). A lymph node excised. Cut surface of the lymph node reveals pale yellow, irregular/serpiginous area, involving a substantial portion of the lymph node which is confirmed microscopically to be a necrotizing (caseating) granulomatous lymphadenitis consistent with *Tuberculous lymphadenitis*

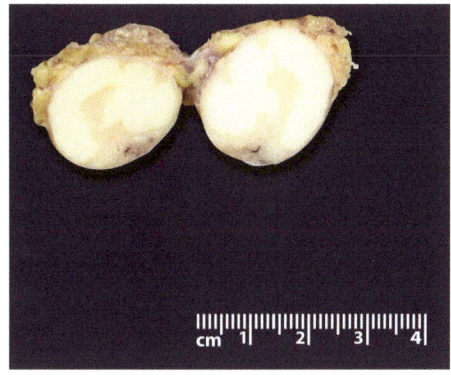

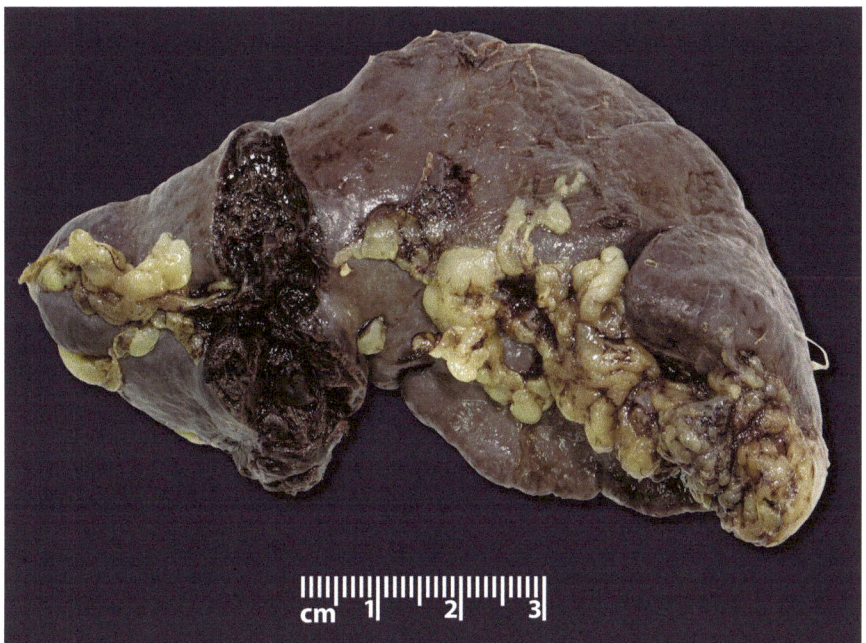

Fig. 9.21 A 44-year-old male underwent splenectomy after a road traffic accident. There is a 4.0 cm laceration associated with a subcapsular hematoma

Fig. 9.22 A 41-year-old male with painless soft tissue swelling in his back. Excision shows a *lipoma*. Notice the smooth surface of the mass covered by a delicate capsule. Cut surface is uniformly yellow (not shown)

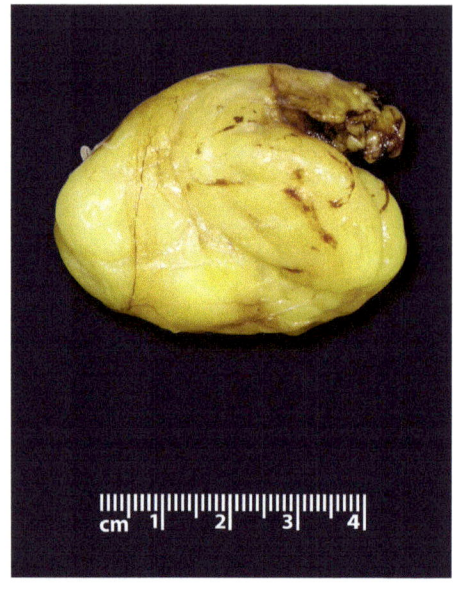

Fig. 9.23 An 80-year-old male with a scalp nodule. Exisional biopsy shows a firm exophytic lesion (0.4 cm in diameter). Microscopically proven to be a *well-differentiated squamous cell carcinoma*

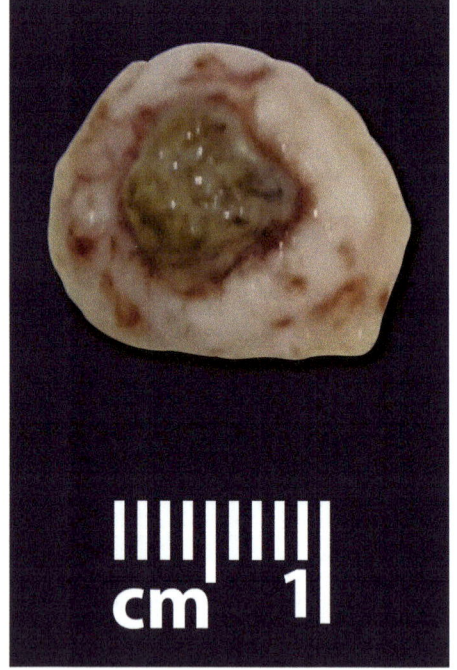

Further Reading

Lester SC. Manual of surgical pathology: expert consult. 3rd ed. Philadelphia: Elsevier/Saunders; 2010.

Part IV

Specimen's 'Essentials'!

Formalin

João Palma

Objective

- Learn about the characteristics of formalin and why formalin is generally considered as the "all-round" tissue fixative.

J. Palma (✉)
Pathology Department, Hospital Vila Franca de Xira, Lisbon, Portugal
e-mail: joao.palma@hvfx.pt

FORMALIN, THE ALL ROUND FIXATIVE!
PART 1

WHY DO WE FIX TISSUE?

In Histopathology most tissues are fixed before being microscopically analysed.

The histological fixation mechanism aims **to stabilize the proteins contained in the tissues to provide resistance to further changes, keeping the cellular architecture and the biomolecular content close to its in vivo state.** Denaturation of tissue proteins, provided by the fixatives, **prevents the activity of putrefaction and autolysis.**

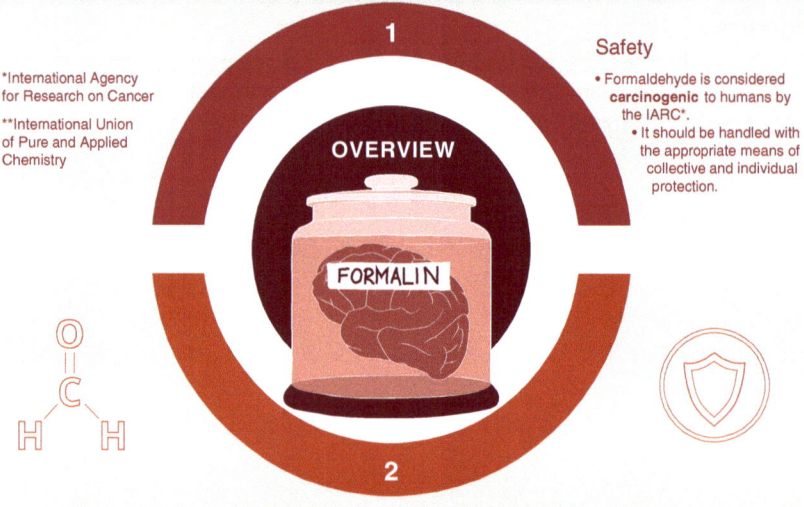

*International Agency for Research on Cancer

**International Union of Pure and Applied Chemistry

1

OVERVIEW

Safety
• Formaldehyde is considered **carcinogenic** to humans by the IARC*.
   • It should be handled with the appropriate means of collective and individual protection.

2

COMPOSITION / ADVANTAGES

• 4% buffered neutral formaldehyde or **10% buffered neutral formalin**

• H2CO – Methanal (IUPAC**)

• Additive non-coagulant fixative

• Connects protein chains, forming bridges

• Penetrates tissue quickly, but fixates slowly

• **Relatively inexpensive and stable**

• **Allows for more special staining techniques than other fixatives**

FORMALIN, THE ALL ROUND FIXATIVE!
PART 2

FACTORS AFFECTING FIXATION

Poor fixation compromises all future work as it is impossible to reconstruct poorly preserved tissue. Several factors affect the quality of fixation.

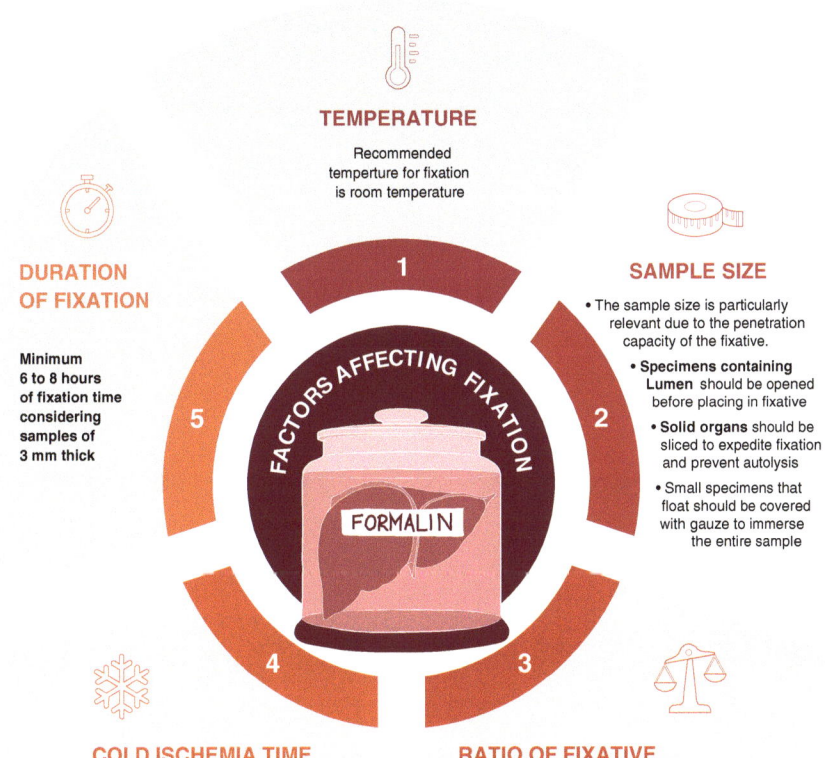

TEMPERATURE

Recommended temperture for fixation is room temperature

DURATION OF FIXATION

Minimum 6 to 8 hours of fixation time considering samples of 3 mm thick

SAMPLE SIZE

- The sample size is particularly relevant due to the penetration capacity of the fixative.
- **Specimens containing Lumen** should be opened before placing in fixative
- **Solid organs** should be sliced to expedite fixation and prevent autolysis
- Small specimens that float should be covered with gauze to immerse the entire sample

FACTORS AFFECTING FIXATION

FORMALIN

COLD ISCHEMIA TIME

Sample is ideally placed in fixative immediately after surgical removal (no more than one hour later)

RATIO OF FIXATIVE VOLUME / SAMPLE SIZE

Fixative volume added to sample should be 15 to 20 times larger than sample volume

Further Reading

Carson FL, Cappellano CH. Histotechnology: a self-instructional text. 4th ed. Chicago: ASCP Press; 2015.

Eltoum I, Fredenburgh J, Myers RB, Grizzle WE. Introduction to the theory and practice of fixation of tissues. J Histotechnol. 2001;24(3):173–90.

Favre HA, Powell WH. Nomenclature of organic chemistry: IUPAC recommendations and preferred names 2013. Cambridge: Royal Society of Chemistry; 2014.

Grizzle WE. The use of fixatives in diagnostic pathology. J Histotechnol. 2001;24(3):151–2.

International Agency for Research on Cancer. Formaldehyde, 2-Butoxyethanol and 1-tert-Butoxypropan-2-ol/IARC Working Group on the Evaluation of Carcinogenic Risks to Humans. Vol. 88. 2004.

Suvarna SK, Layton C, Bancroft JD. Bancroft's theory and practice of histological techniques. Oxford: Elsevier; 2018.

Torlakovic EE, Riddell R, Banerjee D, El-Zimaity H, Pilavdzic D, Dawe P, et al. Canadian Association of Pathologists–Association canadienne des pathologistes National Standards Committee/Immunohistochemistry. Am J Clin Pathol. 2010;133(3):354–65.

Wolff A, Hammond M, Hicks D, Dowsett M, McShane L, Allison K, et al. Recommendations for human epidermal growth factor receptor 2 testing in breast cancer: American Society of Clinical Oncology/College of American Pathologists clinical practice guideline update. J Clin Oncol. 2013;31(31):3997–4013.

The Paraffin Block

11

João Palma

Objectives

Learn about:

- The composition and function of paraffin wax
- The role of paraffin block in tissue embedding and retention
- The proper way for paraffin block storage

J. Palma (✉)
Pathology Department, Hospital Vila Franca de Xira, Lisbon, Portugal
e-mail: joao.palma@hvfx.pt

A. Altaleb (ed.), *Surgical Pathology*,
https://doi.org/10.1007/978-3-030-53690-9_11

73

THE PARAFFIN BLOCK
WHERE THE TISSUE RESTS IN PEACE!
PART 1

OVERVIEW

After dehydration and clearing, the tissue should be impreg -
nated with an appropriate support medium, which is
commonly referred as the **embedding medium**. It allows
hardness to maintain cellular architecture, while obtaining
very thin sections on microtome.

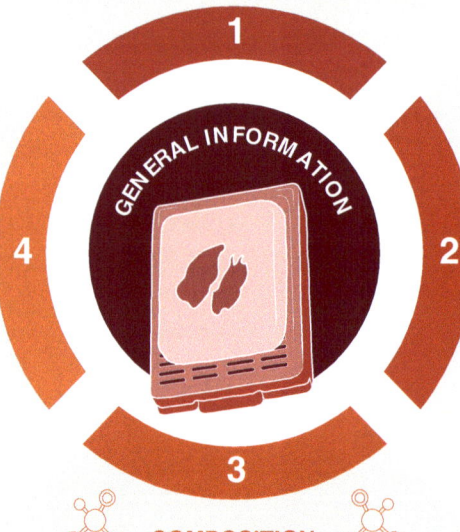

1

2

3

4

GENERAL INFORMATION

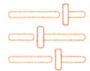

CHARACTER-ISTICS

- Most paraffin waxes for histology melt at **52 – 58°C**
- Should be kept about 2°C above melting point
- Above 60°C could degrade its additives and over harden tissue

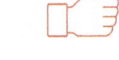

ADVANTAGES

Paraffin wax is **the most used embedding medium** because:

- A large number of tissue blocks can be processed in a relative-ly short time
- Ribboning are effort -lessly obtained
- Routine and most special staining tech-niques can easily be done

COMPOSITION

- Paraffin is a quite inert **combination of hydrocarbons,** produced by the breakage of petroleum
- **Commercial paraffin, sold for tissue embedding, contains various additives such as beeswax, rubber, plastics or dimethylsulphoxide**
- Additives enhance the ability of paraffin to provide adequate support for hard tissues

THE PARAFFIN BLOCK
WHERE THE TISSUE RESTS IN PEACE!

PART 2

EMBEDDING

- Enclosing the tissue in the infiltration medium used for processing and then allowed to solidify
- Specimen orientation is a critical step in embedding
- After embedding in paraffin, the tissue blocks should be cooled rapidly
- All tissue blocks should be identified with a unique patient specimen number, usually generated by pathology LIS, and a second patient identifier

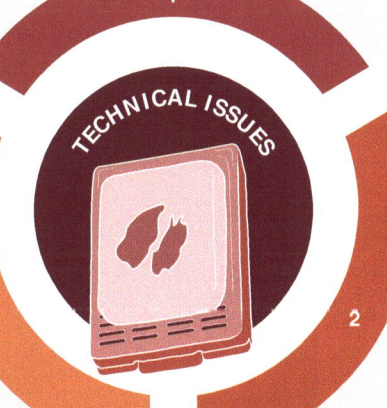

TECHNICAL ISSUES

STORAGE

- The paraffin block archives **should be at room tempera - ture in a location with no direct sun exposure, no significant tempera - ture fluctuations and restricted access**
- When material is trans - ferred between institutions: take special care to minimise the risk of loss
- The temperature during transporta - tion should never reach high values
- **In hot climates, refrigeration may be recom - mended to transport paraffin blocks between institutions**

RETENTION

CAP recommendations:

- Retention of the surgical pathology paraffin blocks during the minimum time of ten years
- Can be longer when required for patient care, education, or quality improvement

The RCP and the IBS (United Kingdom) **recommendations:**

- **Storage of paraffin blocks for at least 30 years, if facilities permit**
- If not, review need for retention every ten years
- Consider for permanent retention: blocks representing rare diseases, known diseases, or thought to have an inherited genetic predisposition
- Alternative to destruction: transfer to an HTA-licensed research biobank

Fig. 11.1 The paraffin block. An embedded piece of tissue is apparent. Notice the information printed on the cassette including case number, pathology laboratory name, and the barcode

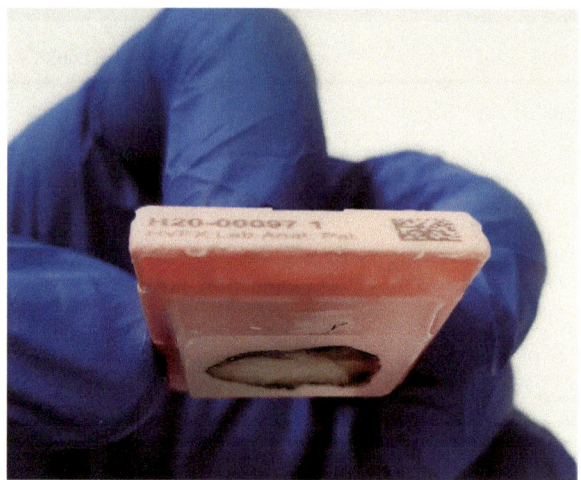

Fig. 11.2 The process of tissue embedding

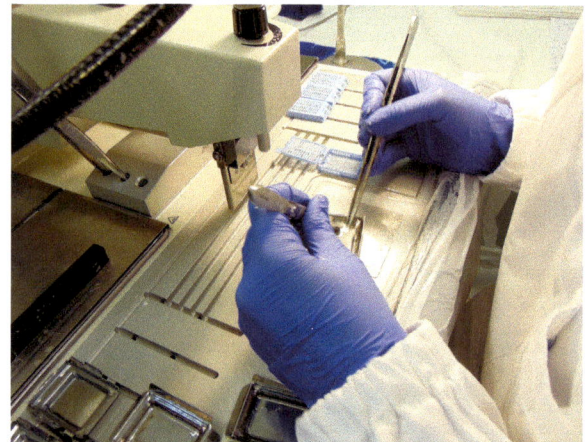

Fig. 11.3 The process of microtomy; delicate tissue sections (as thin as 3–4 μm) can be obtained using this machine

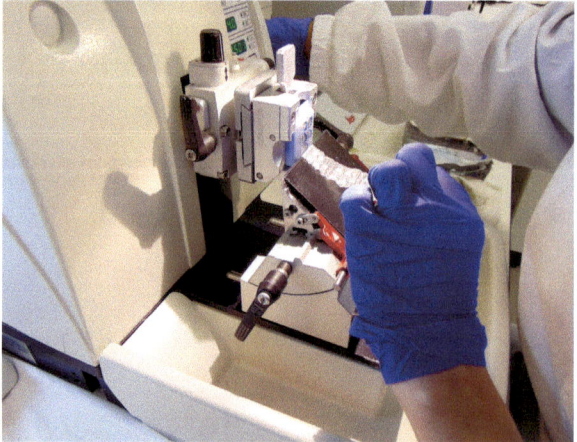

Fig. 11.4 Paraffin blocks archiving/storing. These can be retrieved and new sections can be cut and stained (provided that residual tissue exists within the block). Duration of paraffin blocks retention may vary depending on the institution's policy

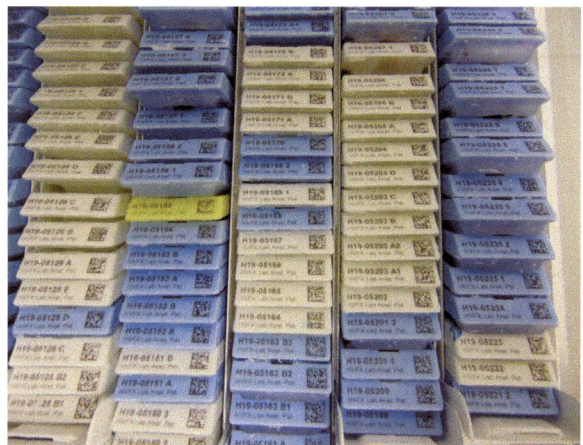

Further Reading

Carson FL, Cappellano CH. Histotechnology: a self-instructional text. 4th ed. Chicago: ASCP Press; 2015.

College of American Pathologists (CAP). Retention of ... [Internet]. cap.org. [Cited 2020]. 2020. https://www.ncleg.gov/documentsites/committees/PMC-LRC2011/December 5, 2012/College of American Pathologist Retention Policy.pdf.

Suvarna SK, Layton C, Bancroft JD. Bancroft's theory and practice of histological techniques. Oxford: Elsevier; 2018.

The retention and storage of pathological records and ... [Internet]. rcpath.org. [Cited 2020]. 2020. https://www.rcpath.org/resourceLibrary/the-retention-and-storage-of-pathological-records-and-specimens%2D%2D5th-edition-.html.

Part V

The Intraoperative Consultation

Ali Lairy and Khaled Alyaqout

Objective

- Learn the role of pathologist in assisting the surgeon intraoperatively by proper clinical collaboration with the surgeon, from a surgeon's point of view.

The study of pathology can be traced back in time to the ancient Greek era. Afterward, it was most notably developed during the golden age of the Islamic era; predominantly through advancing research (Huff 2017; Von Staden 1992; Marketos and Skiadas 1999). However, what we have defined as "modern pathology" may arguably had begun in the second half of the 19th century (Gal 2001). The "frozen section" emerged in the late nineteenth century and was depicted to have an essential role in the 1920s (Taxy 2009; Bloodgood 1927). However, due to the current advances in imaging and modern techniques in biopsies, the role of a pathologist in the operating room has relatively regressed. Nevertheless, indications exist; where an intraoperative consultation of the pathologist may prove invaluable.

The intraoperative role of the pathologist is to provide information that may alter the course of the ongoing surgical procedure (Connolly et al. 2003). The pathologist can guide the surgeon in various ways depending on the indication of the consultation.

For instance, the pathologist may give insight into whether a tumor is benign or malignant. This can significantly alter how radical the surgery being performed is. Take, for example, a cystic lesion on the ovary proves malignant after assessment, necessitating more extensive surgery intraoperatively (Jaafar 2006; Brender et al. 2005).

A. Lairy
Surgical Department, Mubarak Al Kabeer Hospital, Ministry of Health, Jabriya, Kuwait

K. Alyaqout (✉)
Surgical Department, Jaber Al-Ahmad Hospital, South Surra, Kuwait

Furthermore, the pathologist can also aid in the decision to confirm the diagnosis and avoid unnecessary reoperation. This is commonly the case in the excision of a parathyroid adenoma due to hypercalcemia. The removal of the wrong tissue without confirmation would mean that the patient requires a trip back to the operating theater if the correct diagnosis is not confirmed intraoperatively (Jaafar 2006). A gesture the modern-day patient may not appreciate.

Another way of guiding the surgeon is to assess the margin status of a tumor to determine the adequacy of the excision. For example, in squamous cell carcinoma of the head and neck, cosmesis is an important factor in the management. The surgeon will want to be as conservative as possible to provide optimal cosmetic results, while simultaneously not compromising on complete oncological resection (Taxy 2009; Jaafar 2006).

In a more delicate case; a surgeon decides to undertake an excisional biopsy of a suspicious lesion. This lesion is fundamental in determining the diagnosis, yet the location carries a high risk of injury to vital structures (i.e., the root of the mesentery). The presence of an intraoperative pathologist providing input will aid in preventing further risk from unnecessary sampling or the need for reintervention in case of inadequacy (Jaafar 2006).

A vital role for the pathologist is the communication of the information that is requested clearly, with limited jargon, for the surgeon to decide on whether to alter the course of surgery (Connolly et al. 2003; Somerset and Kleinschmidt-DeMasters 2011). For the aforementioned to happen, there need to be certain conditions that are met by both the pathologists and the surgeon.

First, an elective intraoperative consultation would be preferable, and the case is discussed between the pathologist and the surgeon to give adequate time for the pathologist to prepare beforehand (Jaafar 2006).

Next, there must be a valid indication for the intraoperative consultation. The pathologist has the final say in honoring the request or turning it down as an intraoperative frozen section. For example, a lesion that is too small might need to be frozen in its entirety, which would cause distortion of the tissue, and therefore would hinder the more definitive paraffin technique (Taxy 2009; Connolly et al. 2003; Jaafar 2006; Kufe et al. 2003).

Finally, the pathologists must be clear on what is the question that is being asked of them, which part of the body is the sample from, and how to communicate with the surgeon. In addition, pathologists should be aware of their limitations and not to shy away from asking for help from other pathology subspecialties when needed. The pathologist should also be aware of the patient's history and the results of any investigations, including previous pathology slides (Taxy 2009).

References

Bloodgood JC. When cancer becomes a microscopic disease, there must be tissue diagnosis in the operating room. J Am Med Assoc. 1927;88(13):1022–3.
Brender E, Burke A, Glass RM. Frozen section biopsy. JAMA. 2005;294(24):3200.

Connolly JL, Schnitt SJ, Wang HH, Longtine JA, Dvorak A, Dvorak HF. Role of the surgical pathologist in the diagnosis and management of the cancer patient. In: Holland-Frei cancer medicine. 6th ed. Hamilton: BC Decker; 2003.

Gal AA. In search of the origins of modern surgical pathology. Adv Anat Pathol. 2001;8(1):1–3.

Huff TE. The rise of early modern science: Islam, China, and the West. Cambridge: Cambridge University Press; 2017.

Jaafar H. Intra-operative frozen section consultation: concepts, applications and limitations. Malays J Med Sci. 2006;13(1):4.

Kufe DW, Pollock RE, Weichselbaum RR, Bast RC, Gansler TS, Holland JF, Frei E, Connolly JL, Schnitt SJ, Wang HH. Role of the surgical pathologist in the diagnosis and management of the cancer patient. Cancer medicine 6th ed. Hamilton, Ont: BC Decker. 2003.

Marketos SG, Skiadas P. Hippocrates: the father of spine surgery. Spine. 1999;24(13):1381.

Somerset HL, Kleinschmidt-DeMasters BK. Approach to the intraoperative consultation for neurosurgical specimens. Adv Anat Pathol. 2011;18(6):446–9.

Taxy JB. Frozen section and the surgical pathologist: a point of view. Arch Pathol Lab Med. 2009;133(7):1135–8.

Von Staden H. The discovery of the body: human dissection and its cultural contexts in ancient Greece. Yale J Biol Med. 1992;65(3):223.

Intraoperative Diagnoses Techniques

13

Ahmad Altaleb

Objective

- Learn about the different techniques that are utilized by the pathologist to render an intraoperative diagnosis

The main purpose of intraoperative pathologist consultation is to guide immediate surgical management, which can provide surgeons with important information that may be used to modify or even terminate a surgical procedure.

Intraoperative diagnoses are divided into microscopic methods of assessment (e.g., frozen sections) and non-microscopic, that is, gross methods (Fig. 13.1).

Normally, the turnaround time for a single uncomplicated frozen section should not exceed 20 min from the time the specimen is received in the laboratory.

The turnaround time for intraoperative diagnosis depends on:

1. The type of test performed
2. The number of samples/sections submitted for frozen sections
3. The complexity of the specimen (multiple organs/complex anatomy, need for inking multiple margins)

In general, gross examination alone consumes less time than microscopy, and cytologic preparations require less time than frozen sections. Combining these techiques, in the proper settings, can improve the intraoperative diagnostic yield.

A. Altaleb (✉)
Histopathology Department, Mubarak Alkabeer Hospital, Jabriya, Kuwait

© The Editor(s) (if applicable) and The Author(s), under exclusive license
to Springer Nature Switzerland AG 2021
A. Altaleb (ed.), *Surgical Pathology*,
https://doi.org/10.1007/978-3-030-53690-9_13

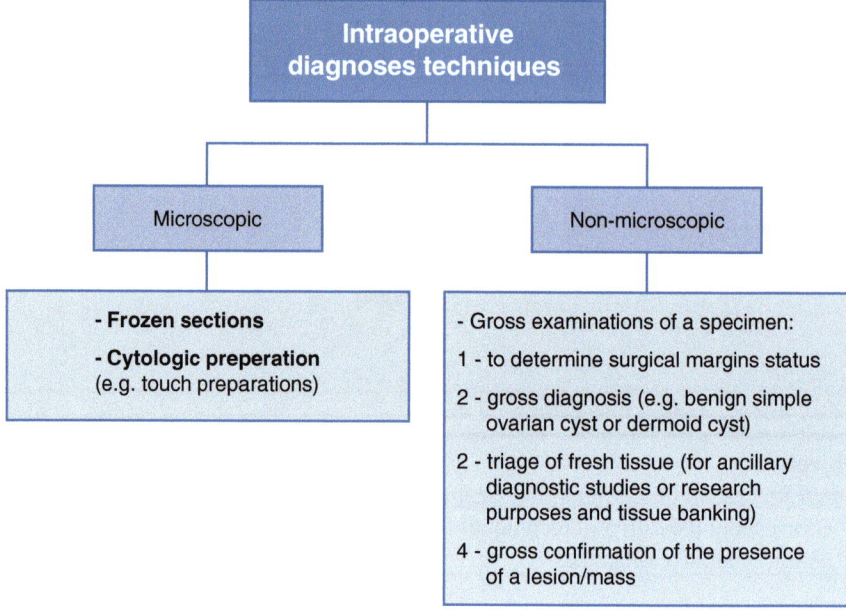

Fig. 13.1 Types of intraoperative diagnoses

Further Reading

Mahe E, Ara S, Bishara M, Kurian A, Tauqir S, Ursani N, et al. Intraoperative pathology consultation: error, cause and impact. Can J Surg. 2013;56(3):E13–8.

Pfeifer JD, Humphrey PA, Ritter JH, Dehner LP. The Washington manual of surgical pathology. Philadelphia: Wolters Kluwer; 2020.

Weidner N. Modern surgical pathology. Philadelphia: Saunders/Elsevier; 2009.

Frozen Sections

14

Ahmad Altaleb

Objective

- Learn about the role of frozen sections during the time of operation, its procedure, and indications.

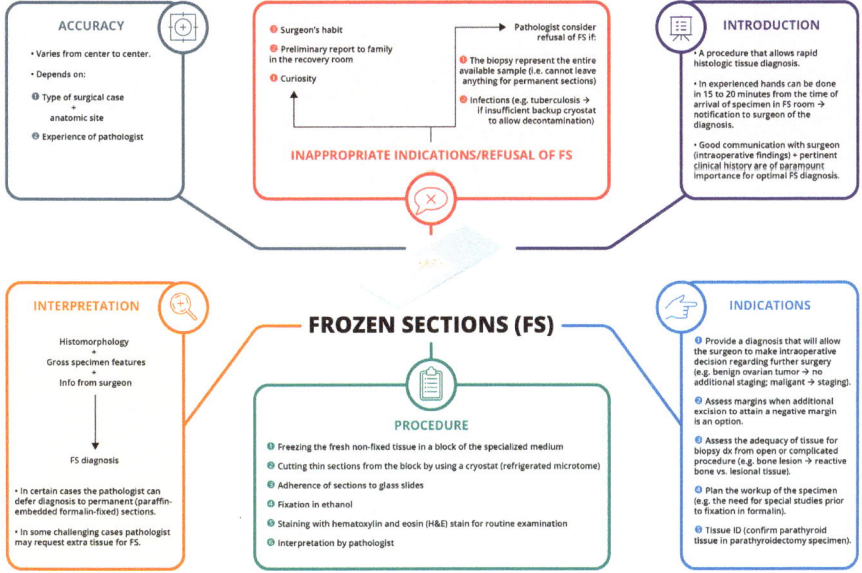

A. Altaleb (✉)
Histopathology Department, Mubarak Alkabeer Hospital, Jabriya, Kuwait

Further Reading

Pfeifer JD, Humphrey PA, Ritter JH, Dehner LP. The Washington manual of surgical pathology. Philadelphia: Wolters Kluwer; 2020.
Weidner N. Modern surgical pathology. Philadelphia: Saunders/Elsevier; 2009.

Part VI

The Biopsy

Biopsies in Oncology: Role, Types, and Principles of Optimal Sampling

15

Ahmad Altaleb

Objectives

- Learn the common methods to obtain biopsies and their diagnostic utilities.
- Learn about the general rules for appropriate neoplastic lesion sampling which would help the pathologist to render a more accurate biopsy diagnosis.

A large bulk of surgical pathology practice consists of biopsy samples. There are several types of biopsies with different approaches to obtain each of them (Figs. 15.1 and 15.2). Currently, there is a trend to minimize open surgical biopsies and rely more on image-guided needle biopsies owing to lower rates of complications and hospital stay.

In the era of cancer medicine, biopsies are performed at the time of identifying a neoplastic process to obtain tissue samples, not only for histologic diagnosis but also to guide therapy by evaluation biomarkers in a growing number of malignant neoplasms including melanoma, colorectal, breast and lung cancers.

Biopsies can also be performed at multiple time points in order to detect progression, predict prognosis, and guide next-line therapy.

Other than their role in oncologic management of disease, biopsies also play an increasing role in oncologic clinical trials to develop and validate biomarkers.

Radiologists using image-guidance are now performing majority of the biopsies.

Limitations

- Biopsies not representative of the main lesion (superficial biopsies, areas of necrosis, inflammation, etc.)
- Artifacts (e.g., cauterization and crushing artifacts)

A. Altaleb (✉)
Histopathology Department, Mubarak Alkabeer Hospital, Jabriya, Kuwait

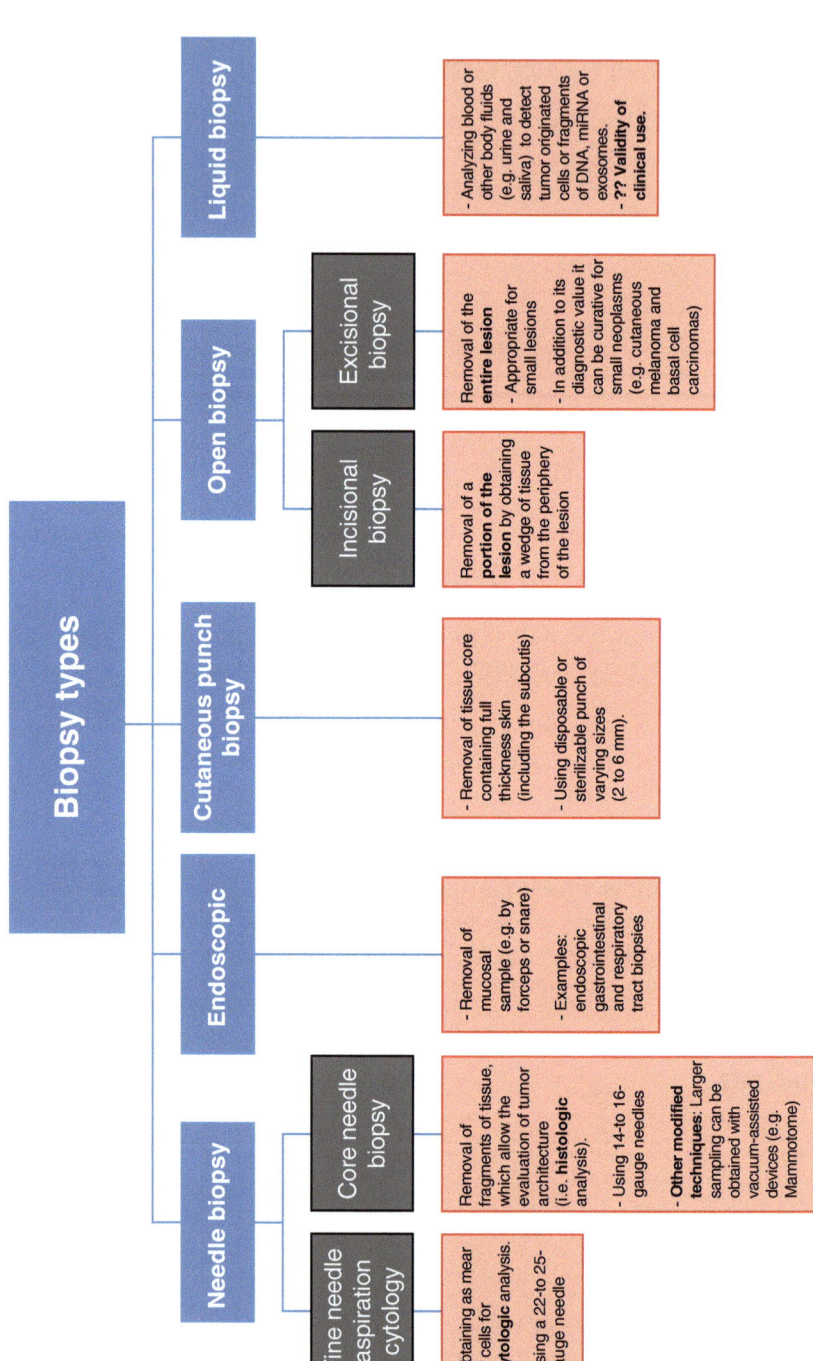

Fig. 15.1 Types of biopsy, general classification

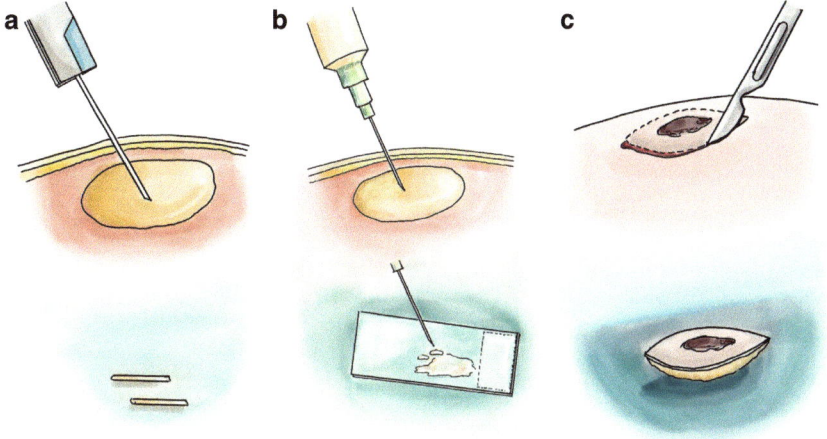

Fig. 15.2 Diagram of some biopsy types: (**a**) core needle biopsy, (**b**) fine needle biopsy, and (**c**) excisional biopsy. (*Illustrations are by lead author Dr. Ahmad Altaleb*)

- Sample fragmentation
- To minimize these limitations and improve the diagnostic yield, there are general rules to follow (Table 15.1).

Potential Competing Alternatives: The Liquid Biopsy

Liquid biopsy offers a noninvasive method to access the tumor by analyzing blood or other body fluids (e.g., urine and saliva) to detect tumor originated cells or fragments of DNA, miRNA, or exosomes. They are emerging as a potential alternative to traditional biopsies.

Three main biomarkers can be accessed through liquid biopsy: circulating tumor cells (CTCs), circulating tumor DNA (ct-DNA), and exosomes containing microRNA.

The advantages of liquid biopsy over tissue biopsy include:

- Rapid and easy to obtain
- Noninvasive
- Lower cost

Possible clinical utilization of liquid biopsies includes:

- Diagnostic purposes
- Identification and tracking of tumor-specific alterations during disease progression
- Guiding therapeutic decisions

In 2016 Food and Drug Administration (FDA) approved two liquid biopsy companion diagnostic tests for EGFR mutation in plasma cell-free tumor DNA (cfDNA) for patients with non-small-cell lung cancer in clinical practice.

Table 15.1 Principles of optimal sampling

Principle	Rationale
If there is a provisional clinical diagnosis this should be mentioned clearly in the request form or communicated to the pathologist	To allow the pathologist to consider any ancillary studies (e.g., flow cytometry in non-Hodgkin lymphoma, cytogenetic/molecular studies, touch imprint cytologic examination)
Try to avoid central ulcerated areas (in ulcerated tumors). The periphery that includes normal and diseased tissue is the most informative area	Ulcerated areas may show only necrosis and inflammation
Avoid squeezing of tissue with forceps	To avoid crushing artifact that may render the biopsy diagnosis difficult
In deep-seated lesions, sometimes, marked peripheral tissue reaction may develop, so the biopsy should not be too peripheral	Tissue reaction may include fibrosis, chronic inflammation, and calcification or even metaplastic bone formation, which may be the only sampled tissue
Try to take more numerous biopsies for large lesions	– Diagnostic foci may be present only focally – Variability in the growth patterns may exists
Try to avoid superficial biopsy/sampling	For proper assessment of the relationship between neoplastic epithelium and stroma (i.e, identify invasive foci)
In case of tissue fragmentation, send all the material to pathology (all of them would be submitted for microscopic examination)	Sometimes grossly less impressive tiny fragment is the one that contains the diagnostic area of interest!
Place the biopsy into a container with the appropriate and adequate fixative (e.g., formalin) and avoid any further manual manipulation of the obtained samples. (N.B. This applies only for specimens that do not require pre-fixation ancillary studies; ask your pathologist if in doubt!)	To avoid and minimize any artifact

However, the integration of liquid biopsies into routine clinical practice remains limited for several reasons including the lack of consensus on the ideal/standardized technical approach and the difficulty in detecting DNA fragments in the blood especially in the early stages of cancer.

Further Reading

Bai Y, Zhao H. Liquid biopsy in tumors: opportunities and challenges. Ann Transl Med. 2018;6(S1):S89.

Ramaswamy G. Washington manual of oncology. 2nd ed. St. Louis: Wolters Kluwer Medical; 2008.

Rosai J. Rosai and Ackerman's surgical pathology. Edinburgh: Mosby; 2011.

Siravegna G, et al. Integrating liquid biopsies into the management of cancer. Nat Rev Clin Oncol. 2017;14:531–48. https://doi.org/10.1038/Nrclinonc.2017.14.

Tam AL, Lim HJ, Wistuba LI, Tamrazi A, Kuo MD, Ziv E, et al. Image-guided biopsy in the era of personalized cancer care: proceedings from the society of interventional radiology research consensus panel. J Vasc Interv Radiol. 2016;27(1):8–19.

Part VII

Ancillary Studies in Surgical Pathology

Ancillary Studies in Surgical Pathology

16

Nicolas Kozakowski

Objective

- Learn the commonly utilized ancillary studies/techniques in surgical pathology (classical and modern ones) and the rationale behind their use.

N. Kozakowski (✉)
Department of Pathology, Medical University of Vienna, Vienna, Austria
e-mail: nicolas.kozakowski@meduniwien.ac.at

ANCILLARY STUDIES
IN SURGICAL PATHOLOGY
PART 1

SUPPLEMENTARY STAININGS
("SPECIAL STAINS")

To identify properties of tissues, cells (or their sub-cellular
components) or the non-cellular parts of a tissue.

Microorganisms

- **Bacteria:** Gram (positive bacteria in violet, negative
  bacteria in pink), Ziehl-Neelsen &
  auramine–rhodamine & Kinyoun acid-fast stains
  (mycobacteria, nocardia), Mucicarmine for
  Cryptococcus, Wharthin-Starry (spirochetes,
  helicobacter), Giemsa (trichomonas,
  spirochetes), Gomori's methenamine
  (pneumocystis), Papanicolaou

- **Viruses:** Giemsa,
  Papanicolaou

- **Fungi:** PAS; Gomori's
  methenamine

Mucins
PAS, Alcian blue, Mucicarmine

Collagen and interstitium
Masson trichrome, AFOG, Sirius red, reticulin

Iron Prussian blue, Perls' blue stain

Elastic fibers Elastica van Gieson

Copper Rhodanine stain

Amyloid substance
Congo red

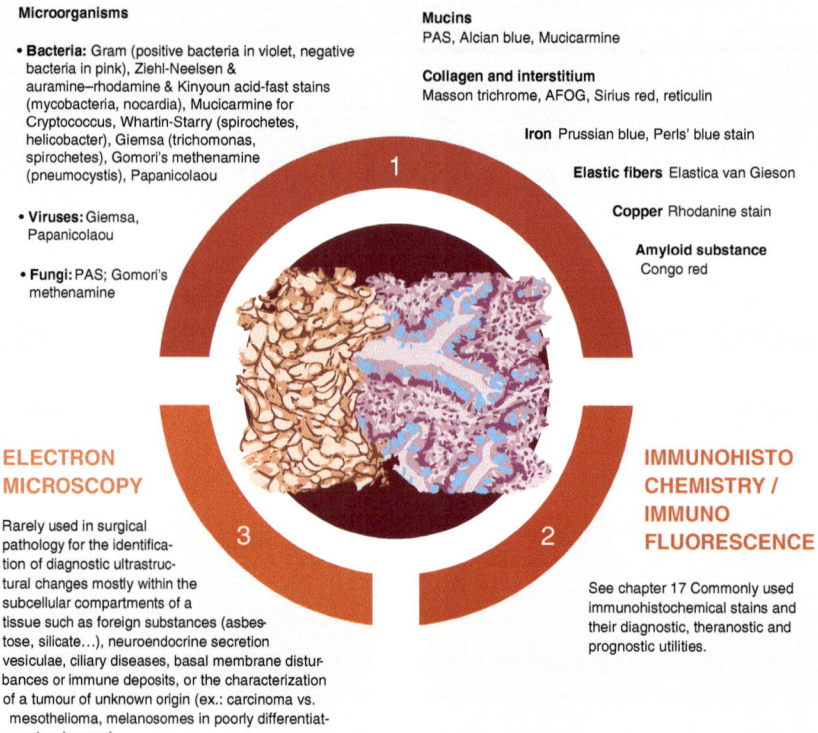

1

ELECTRON
MICROSCOPY

Rarely used in surgical
pathology for the identification of diagnostic ultrastruc-
tural changes mostly within the
subcellular compartments of a
tissue such as foreign substances (asbes-
tose, silicate...), neuroendocrine secretion
vesiculae, ciliary diseases, basal membrane distur-
bances or immune deposits, or the characterization
of a tumour of unknown origin (ex.: carcinoma vs.
mesothelioma, melanosomes in poorly differentiated melanoma)

3

IMMUNOHISTO
CHEMISTRY /
IMMUNO
FLUORESCENCE

See chapter 17 Commonly used
immunohistochemical stains and
their diagnostic, theranostic and
prognostic utilities.

2

ANCILLARY STUDIES
IN SURGICAL PATHOLOGY
PART 2

CYTOGENETICS

Most of these techniques are now available for formalin fixed paraffin embedded tissue but some of them only feasible from frozen material or blood (**talk with your pathologist!**)

• **Karyotype analysis** (for chromosomic rearrangements)
• **Mutation in diverse diseases:** Von Recklinghausen (NF-1 mutation), metabolic disorders, familial cancer disorders (MSI, BRCA1&2, MEN1&2)

• **Sequencing**

Southern blot, PCR, RT-PCR, qPCR, next-generation sequencing (NGS) for the identification of oncogenes and tumour suppressor genes (NRAS, BRAF and cKIT mutations for differential diagnosis or prediction of response to targeted therapy; detection of the diagnosis-specific translocation of diverse tumours (ex.: translocation t (9:22) for chronic myeloid leukemia)), clonality analysis of T-cell neoplasms or the detection of microorganisms (ex.: HPV, mycobacteria, borreliosis, pneumocystis, fungus)

• **MSI analysis (fragment length analysis)**
• **Fluorescent or chromogenic in situ hybridisation (FISH or CISH)**

Detection of the presence or absence of a specific DNA or RNA sequence, often used to confirm findings of immunohistochemistry (mutations (PD-L1, microsatellite instability, HER-2 (ex.: breast cancer), tumor-specific mutations (ex.: Ewing's sarcoma (translocation t(11:22)); synovial sarcoma (translocation (X:18)); haematopoietic neoplasms (ex.: translocation t(14:18) for follicular lymphoma).

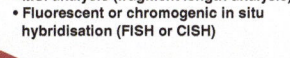

EPIGENETICS

Methylation status
Colon carcinoma

Tumour suppressors
p16 protein of gene CDKN2A for squamous cell carcinomas of diverse localisation; p53 for solid tissue cancer, melanoma or hematopoietic cancer

Microsatellite instability
MLH1, MSH2, MSH6 and PMS2 in colon carcinoma

IMMUNOHISTO CHEMISTRY

Targets of immunotherapy
PD-L1 for lung or urothelial carcinoma, EGFR-mutation for the prediction of response to anti-EGFR targeted therapy

Oncogenes
cKIT for melanoma or soft tissue tumours

Further Reading

Böcker W, Denk H, Heitz PU, et al. Lehrbuch Pathologie. Amsterdam: Elsevier Health Sciences; 2019.

Ilyas M. Next-generation sequencing in diagnostic pathology. Pathobiology. 2017;84(6):292–305.

Makki JS. Diagnostic implication and clinical relevance of ancillary techniques in clinical pathology practice. Clin Med Insights Pathol. 2016;9:5–11.

Netto GJ, Saad RD. Diagnostic molecular pathology: an increasingly indispensable tool for the practicing pathologist. Arch Pathol Lab Med. 2006;130:1339–48.

Rosai J. Rosai and Ackerman's surgical pathology. Edinburgh: Mosby; 2011.

Werner M, Wilkens L, Aubele M, Nolte M, Zitzelsberger H, Komminoth P. Interphase cytogenetics in pathology: principles, methods, and applications of fluorescence in situ hybridization (FISH). Histochem Cell Biol. 1997;108(4–5):381–90.

Commonly Used Immunohistochemical Stains and Their Diagnostic, Theranostic, and Prognostic Utilities

17

Nicolas Kozakowski

Objective

- Learn the importance of immunohistochemistry as an adjunct study in surgical pathology.

Introduction

Immunohistochemistry is a technique based on antigen–antibody binding reaction. It visualizes the distribution and localization of specific antigen or cellular components in tissue sections.

Based on the affinity of mono- or polyclonal antibodies produced in variable species (mostly mouse, rabbit, or goat) to specifically recognize protein epitopes, it helps in recognizing tissue- or cell-specific proteins and can be applied as a direct, an indirect, or a multistep assay. Most of the time a combination of antibodies ("immunohistochemical profile") is used to confirm a diagnosis.

Diagnostic Use

Organ Diagnosis

- Intestinal differentiation
  CDX2
- Thyroid and lung
  TTF-1

N. Kozakowski (✉)
Department of Pathology, Medical University of Vienna, Vienna, Austria
e-mail: nicolas.kozakowski@meduniwien.ac.at

- Prostate
  PSA, PSA-P
- Lymphoid cells
  CD45
- Melanocytic cells
  Melan-A, HMB45, S-100
- Germ cells and liver
  Alpha-fetoprotein
- Thyroid gland, parathyroid glands, C-cells, beta-islets of the pancreas
  Hormones, hormone receptors and secretory vesicles of neuroendocrine
  (respectively *thyroglobulin, parathormone, calcitonin, insulin, glucagon…*).
- Syncytiotrophoblast
  Beta-HCG

Differentiation

- Epithelial
  Cytokeratin (*CK1 to CK20*, numerated inversely depending on their molecular
  weight and basic or acidic character). A combination of CK of low- and high-
  molecular weight will give an idea on the organ systems from where a tumor
  might come from (e.g., *CK7− and CK20+*: gastrointestinal tract or *CK7+ and
  CK20−*: endometrial origin, biliary tract, mesothelioma).
- Hematopoietic
  Cluster of differentiation (CD): broadly present types of antigen at the surface of
  different hematopoietic cells or subtypes of lymphoproliferative disorders (e.g.,
  CD45 is the common marker of leukocytes). A profile of cluster of differentiation is specific to certain subtypes of leukocytes; Pan-T-cells antigens: *CD3,
  CD5*; Pan-B-cells antigens: *CD20, CD79a*. Clonality of B-cells: *kappa and
  lambda light-chains*. Clusters of differentiation are not only present in hemato-
  poietic cells (e.g., *CD56 (or NCAM)* is expressed in some lymphomas but also
  neuroendocrine tumor cells).
- Mesenchymal
  Vimentin: a common marker of mesenchymal differentiation. It can be encoun-
  tered in other neoplasms such as melanoma, renal cell carcinoma, and
  mesothelioma.
- Neural
  S-100, GFAP.
- Muscular
  Smooth muscle actin; desmin (striated fibers).
- Vascular
  Endothelial (*CD31, CD34, Factor VIII*).
- Melanocytic
  Melan-*A; HMB45* (naevus cells or melanoma).
- Neuroendocrine
  Hormones, hormone receptors, and secretory vesicles of neuroendocrine organs
  or (sometimes secreting) tumors (*thyroglobulin, parathormone, calcitonin, insu-
  lin, glucagon, or ACTH* …), tumors with neuroendocrine differentiation (*chro-
  mogranin A, synaptophysin, CD56*).

Inflammation

- Immune deposits
  Immunoglobulins and complement in inflammatory diseases (e.g., *IgG4* in IgG4-associated inflammatory diseases).
- Subtyping of infiltrating leukocytes
  CD3 or CD5: T-cells
  CD20: B-cells
  CD38 and CD138: plasma cells

Tumor Subtypes

- Mammary carcinoma
  E-Cadherin (+: ductal; −: lobular).
- Lung/Pleura malignant tumor
  CK7, napsin, EMA, Ber-EP4, TTF-1 (adenocarcinoma) versus *CK5/6, p63* (squamous cell carcinoma) versus *calretinin, CK5/6, mesothelin, thrombomodulin, WT-1* (mesothelioma).
- Ovarian carcinoma
  CA125.
- Gastrointestinal and biliopancreatic carcinoma
  CA19-9.
- Intestinal adenocarcinoma
  CDX-2.
- Adenocarcinoma (vs. other carcinomas)
  CEA.
- Squamous cell carcinoma
  CK5/6, p63.
- Prostatic carcinoma
  PSA, PSA-P.
- GIST
  cKIT, DOG1.
- Adipocytic tumors
  MDM2; CDK4 in well-differentiated and dedifferentiated liposarcoma.

Infections

- Bacterial
  Helicobacter pylori; Mycobacterium tuberculosis; Tropheryma *whipplei*; *rickettsia sp.*; *bartonella sp.*; *borellia sp.*; *Treponema pallidum*; *staphylococcus sp.*; *streptococcus sp.*; *clostridium sp.*; *Escherichia coli*.
- Viral
  HSV 1 and 2 (herpes simplex viruses); *CMV* (cytomegalovirus); *EBV* (Epstein–Barr virus); *BK-virus* (Polyomavirus); *HPV* (human papilloma viruses); *HHV* (human herpes viruses); *adenovirus, parvovirus B19*; *VZV* (varicella zoster virus); *Hepatitis B or C viruses*.
- Fungal and parasitic
  Candida sp., Aspergillus sp.; *Cryptococcus neoformans*; *Pneumocystis carinii*

– Protozoan
  Leishmania; *Toxoplasma gondii*; *trichomonas Vaginalis*; *Trypanosomia sp.*;
  Entamoeba histolytica; *Giarda lamblia*

Theranostic Use

The immunohistochemical detection of the following proteins supports the decision
for hormonal deprivation or targeted therapy.

– Lung adenocarcinoma
  EGFR, ALK, cMET, ROS1, PD-L1
– Breast carcinoma
  *Estrogen and progesterone receptors, BRCA1&2, HER2, PI3K/AKT, androgen
  receptor*
– Colon adenocarcinoma
  EGFR, VEGF, VEGFR, KRAS, NRAS, BRAF
– Gastric adenocarcinoma
  HER2, VEGF, VEGFR, EGFR, c-MET, mTOR
– Prostatic adenocarcinoma
  PDGFR, HER2, VEGF
– Melanoma
  BRAF V600E, NRAS, PD-L1
– Ovarian carcinoma
  VEGFR, PDGFR, BRCA1&2, PD-L1
– Renal cell carcinoma
  VEGFR, EGFR; PDGFR, HER2, PD-L1
– GIST
  cKIT, PDGFR-A

Prognostic Use

– Proliferation marker
  Ki-67 is in many tumors a marker of poor prognosis (gastric, pulmonary; pros-
  tatic adenocarcinoma)
– Cell cycle markers
  Cyclin D-1, p16INK4 in melanoma
– Oncogenes
  HER2 in mammary, pulmonary or colorectal carcinoma
  Bcl-2 in melanoma
  cKIT in GIST, lung adenocarcinoma, melanoma
  BRAF in thyroid papillary carcinoma, melanoma, colorectal carcinoma, lung
  carcinoma
  cMET and HGF in testicular tumors
– Tumor suppressors

p53 is in many tumors a marker of poor prognosis (gastric carcinoma; lung adenocarcinoma; prostate carcinoma)

BRCA1 and 2 in breast carcinoma

PTEN in prostatic adenocarcinoma
- Vascular and lymphatic markers
  CD31, CD34, podoplanin in melanoma (better detection of angio- or lymphangioinvasion)
- DNA mismatch repair
  Microsatellite instability syndrome in colon carcinoma (*MSH6, MSH2, MLH1, PMS2*)
- Neuroendocrine differentiation
  Worse prognosis for prostatic adenocarcinoma
- Hormone receptors
  Androgen receptor for prostatic carcinoma
  Estrogen- or progesterone receptors in breast cancer

Further Reading

Bellizzi AM. Immunohistochemistry in the diagnosis and classification of neuroendocrine neoplasms: what can brown do for you? Hum Pathol. 2020;96:8–33.

Eyzaguirre E, Haque AK. Application of immunohistochemistry to infections. Arch Pathol Lab Med. 2008;132:424–31.

Garcia CF, Swerdlow SH. Best practices in contemporary diagnostic immunohistochemistry: panel approach to hematolymphoid proliferations. Arch Pathol Lab Med. 2009;133:756–65.

Ivell R, Teerds K, Hoffman GE. Proper application of antibodies for immunohistochemical detection: antibody crimes and how to prevent them. Endocrinology. 2014;155(3):676–87.

Kaliyappan K, Palanisamy M, Duraiyan J, Govindarajan R. Applications of immunohistochemistry. J Pharm Bioallied Sci. 2012;4(6):307.

Kiyozumi Y, Iwatsuki M, Yamashita K, Koga Y, Yoshida N, Baba H. Update on targeted therapy and immune therapy for gastric cancer, 2018. J Cancer Metastasis Treat. 2018;4(6):31.

Liu C, Ghayouri M, Brown IS. Immunohistochemistry and special stains in gastrointestinal pathology practice. Diagn Histopathol. 2020;26(1):22–32.

Molina-Ruiz AM, Santonja C, Rütten A, Cerroni L, Kutzner H, Requena L. Immunohistochemistry in the diagnosis of cutaneous viral infections—part I. Cutaneous viral infections by herpesviruses and papillomaviruses. Am J Dermatopathol. 2015;37(1):1–14.

Tsutsumi Y. Low-specificity and high-sensitivity immunostaining for demonstrating pathogens in formalin-fixed, paraffin-embedded sections. Immunohistochemistry—The Ageless Biotechnology, Charles F. Streckfus, IntechOpen, https://doi.org/10.5772/intechopen.85055. Available from: https://www.intechopen.com/books/immunohistochemistry-the-ageless-biotechnology/low-specificity-and-high-sensitivity-immunostaining-for-demonstratingpathogens-in-formalin-fixed-pa.

Yatabe Y, Dacic S, Borczuk AC, Warth A, Russell PA, Lantuejoul S, et al. Best practices recommendations for diagnostic immunohistochemistry in lung cancer. J Thorac Oncol. 2019;14(3):377–407.

Grading and Staging in Pathology

18

Nicolas Kozakowski

Objective

- Learn the principles of pathologic grading and staging of malignant tumors.

Grading

Classification system of malignant tumors in relation with their differentiation grade.
　It varies depending on the type of tumor and is related to its biological behavior (growth and spreading).

- G1: resembling the original tissue
- G2: intermediate differentiation
- G3: poorly differentiated, with polymorphism, marked anisocytosis and anisokaryosis
- G4: undifferentiated, anaplastic
  There are some tumor-specific grading systems:

- World Health Organization (WHO)/International Society for Urologic Pathology (ISUP) grading system (superseding the Fuhrman grade) of renal cell carcinoma
- Gleason grade of prostatic adenocarcinoma
- Nottingham grading system of breast cancer
- Fédération Nationale des Centres de Lutte Contre Le Cancer (FNCLCC) system or National Cancer Institute (NCI) of soft tissue sarcomas
- WHO grading system of brain tumor

N. Kozakowski (✉)
Department of Pathology, Medical University of Vienna, Vienna, Austria
e-mail: nicolas.kozakowski@meduniwien.ac.at

A. Altaleb (ed.), *Surgical Pathology*,
https://doi.org/10.1007/978-3-030-53690-9_18

109

Staging

The classification system of malignant tumors is in relation with their local (organ), locoregional (growth over the organ limits, to the vascular or lymphatic structures or the lymph nodes in the vicinity of the tumor), and distant extent (metastasis). It is applied to determine the prognosis of the neoplastic disease and support therapy decision.

The most used staging system is the organ-specific TNM system, generated by the American Joint Committee on Cancer (AJCC) and the Union for International Cancer Control (UICC) and based on the size and local extent of the Tumor ("T"), its extent to loco-regional lymph Nodes ("N"), and the presence of distant Metastasis ("M"). The kind of assessment is taken into account, with the addition of a prefix written in a minuscule letter. It indicates whether a pathologist ("p") or a clinician ("c") evaluated the staging. As well, a status post-therapy ("y"), retreatment ("r"), or a diagnosis made at autopsy time ("a") can be acknowledged. Furthermore, the site of metastasis can be specified (e.g., PUL for lung and HEP for liver).

(See Chap. 20.)

Other organ-specific staging systems:

- International Federation of Gynecology and Obstetrics (FIGO) staging system for vulvar, cervical, or endometrial cancer
- Dukes staging system for colorectal cancer
- Clark level and Breslow depth for melanoma
- Ann Arbor staging system for Hodgkin lymphoma
  Some of them have been modified and adapted to tumor subtypes.

Further Reading

Böcker W, Denk H, Heitz PU, et al. Lehrbuch Pathologie. Amsterdam: Elsevier Health Sciences; 2019.

A Primer on Clinical Stage Classifications of Malignant Tumors (cTNM)

Ahmad Altaleb

Objective

• Learn the principles of clinical staging of malignant tumors.

Staging a tumor is an anatomical exercise that uses a combination of clinical examination and radiology/imaging.

The most clinically useful staging system is the tumor, node, and metastasis (TNM) staging system developed by the American Joint Committee on Cancer (AJCC) in collaboration with the Union for International Cancer Control (UICC).

This staging system is based on:

1. The primary **t**umor (size/extent) = T
2. The presence of regional lymph **n**ode metastases = N
3. Distant **m**etastases = M

Classification of T, N, and M during the diagnostic workup time frame is denoted by the use of a lower case c prefix: cT, cN, and cM0, cM1 or pM1 (or the use of no prefix: T, N, M).

As a general rule, T0 indicates no visible evidence of primary tumor, while T1–4 indicates an increasing degree of local tumor extent. Likewise, N0 means regional lymph nodes are negative for metastasis, while N1–3 indicates an increasing involvement of regional nodes.

M0 indicates no distant metastases whereas M1 indicates the presence of metastases. Last, Nx and Mx mean that the lymph nodes and distant metastases cannot be assessed, respectively.

A. Altaleb (✉)
Histopathology Department, Mubarak Alkabeer Hospital, Jabriya, Kuwait

Clinical stage is important to record for all patients:

1. For selecting initial therapy.
2. For comparison across patient cohorts when some have surgery as a component of initial treatment and others do not.

Time frame:
Clinical classification is based on information gathered about the extent of cancer from the time of diagnosis until the initiation of primary treatment or the decision for watchful waiting or supportive care, and is based on the shorter of two periods of time:

• Within 4 months after diagnosis, or
• The time of cancer progression (if cancer progresses before the end of the 4-month window)

Criteria:
All patients with cancer identified before treatment.
Components of the diagnostic workup (Fig. 19.1):

Notes

• The tumor must have a diagnostic workup including at least a history and physical examination to assign a clinical stage. The managing physician (usually a surgical or medical oncologist) gathers data from multiple sources to assign a clinical stage.

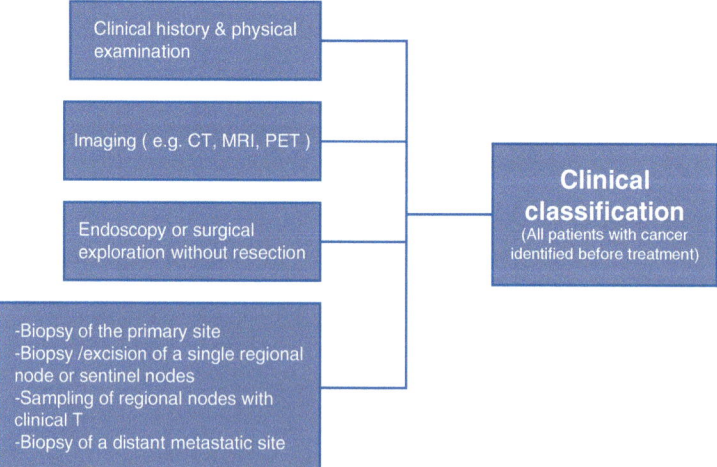

Fig. 19.1 Components of the diagnostic workup that should be considered while assigning a clinical stage (cTNM)

- Imaging is important despite the fact it is not necessary to assign a clinical stage.
- The clinical stage may be the only stage classification by which comparisons can be made across all patients, because not all patients will undergo surgical treatment before other therapy, and response to treatment varies.

Further Reading

Adam A, Dixon AK, Gillard JH, Schaefer-Prokop C, Grainger RG, Allison DJ. Grainger & Allison's diagnostic radiology e-book. London: Churchill Livingstone; 2014.
Amin MB. AJCC cancer staging manual. Chicago: American College of Surgeons; 2018.
Bower M, Waxman J. Lecture notes: oncology. Chichester: Wiley; 2017.

Selected Tables of Pathologic Stage Classification (pTNM)

Ahmad Altaleb

Objective

- Learn and familiarize yourself with some examples of the pathologic TNM staging systems.

Major salivary glands tumors pathologic staging

T category	T criteria
TX	Primary tumor cannot be assessed
T0	No evidence of primary tumor
Tis	Carcinoma in situ
T1	Tumor 2 cm or smaller in greatest dimension without extraparenchymal extension
T2	Tumor larger than 2 cm but not larger than 4 cm in greatest dimension without extra parenchymal extension
T3	Tumor larger than 4 cm and/or tumor having an extraparenchymal extension
T4	*Moderately advanced* (tumor invades skin, mandible, ear canal, and/or facial nerve) *or very advanced disease* (tumor invades skull base and/or pterygoid plates and/or encases carotid artery)

N category	N criteria
NX	Regional lymph nodes cannot be assessed
N0	No regional lymph node metastasis
N1	Metastasis in a single ipsilateral lymph node, 3 cm or smaller in greatest dimension and ENE[a](−)

A. Altaleb (✉)
Histopathology Department, Mubarak Alkabeer Hospital, Jabriya, Kuwait

N category	N criteria
N2	Metastasis in a single ipsilateral lymph node, 3 cm or smaller in greatest dimension and ENE(+); *or* larger than 3 cm but not larger than 6 cm in greatest dimension and ENE(−); *or* metastases in multiple ipsilateral lymph node(s), none larger than 6 cm in greatest dimension and ENE(−); *or* in bilateral or contralateral lymph nodes, none larger than 6 cm in greatest dimension and ENE(−)
N3	Metastasis in a lymph node larger than 6 cm in greatest dimension and ENE(−); *or* in a single ipsilateral node larger than 3 cm in greatest dimension and ENE(+); *or* multiple ipsilateral, contralateral, or bilateral nodes any with ENE(+); *or* a single contralateral node of any size and ENE(+)

M category	M criteria
M0	No distant metastasis
M1	Distant metastasis

[a]*ENE* Extranodal Extension

Lung tumors pathologic staging

T category	T criteria
TX	Primary tumor cannot be assessed, or tumor proven by the presence of malignant cells in sputum or bronchial washings but not visualized by imaging or bronchoscopy
T0	No evidence of primary tumor
Tis	Carcinoma in situ
	Squamous cell carcinoma in situ (SCIS) Adenocarcinoma in situ (AIS): adenocarcinoma with a pure lepidic pattern, ≤3 cm in greatest dimension
T1	Tumor ≤ 3 cm in greatest dimension, surrounded by lung or visceral pleura, without bronchoscopic evidence of invasion more proximal than the lobar bronchus (i.e., not in the main bronchus)
T2	Tumor > 3 cm but ≤ 5 cm or having any of the following features: • Involves the main bronchus regardless of the distance to the carina, but without the involvement of the carina • Invades visceral pleura (PL1 or PL2) • Associated with atelectasis or obstructive pneumonitis that extends to the hilar region, involving part or all of the lung T2 tumors with these features are classified as T2a if ≤4 cm or if the size cannot be determined and T2b if >4 cm but ≤5 cm
T3	Tumor >5 cm but ≤7 cm in greatest dimension or directly invading any of the following: parietal pleura (PL3), chest wall (including superior sulcus tumors), phrenic nerve, parietal pericardium; or separate tumor nodule(s) in the same lobe as the primary
T4	Tumor > 7 cm or tumor of any size invading one or more of the following: diaphragm, mediastinum, heart, great vessels, trachea, recurrent laryngeal nerve, esophagus, vertebral body, or carina; separate tumor nodule(s) in an ipsilateral lobe different from that of the primary

N category	N criteria
NX	Regional lymph nodes cannot be assessed
N0	No regional lymph node metastasis
N1	Metastasis in ipsilateral peribronchial and/or ipsilateral hilar lymph nodes and intrapulmonary nodes, including involvement by direct extension
N2	Metastasis in ipsilateral mediastinal and/or subcarinal lymph node(s)
N3	Metastasis in contralateral mediastinal, contralateral hilar, ipsilateral or contralateral scalene, or supraclavicular lymph node(s)

M category	M criteria
M0	No distant metastasis
M1	Distant metastasis
M1a	Separate tumor nodule(s) in a contralateral lobe; tumor with pleural or pericardial nodules or malignant pleural or pericardial effusion. Most pleural (pericardial) effusions with lung cancer are a result of the tumor. In a few patients, however, multiple microscopic examinations of pleural (pericardial) fluid are negative for tumor, and the fluid is non-bloody and not an exudate. If these elements and clinical judgment dictate that the effusion is not related to the tumor, the effusion should be excluded as a staging descriptor
M1b	Single extrathoracic metastasis in a single organ (including involvement of a single nonregional node)
M1c	Multiple extrathoracic metastases in a single organ or multiple organs

Breast carcinoma pathologic staging

T category	T criteria
TX	Primary tumor cannot be assessed
T0	No evidence of primary tumor
Tis (DCIS)	Ductal carcinoma in situ
Tis (Paget)	Paget disease of the nipple NOT associated with invasive carcinoma and/or carcinoma in situ (DCIS) in the underlying breast parenchyma. Carcinomas in the breast parenchyma associated with Paget disease are categorized based on the size and characteristics of the parenchymal disease, although the presence of Paget disease should still be noted
T1	Tumor $\leq$ 20 mm in greatest dimension
T2	Tumor > 20 mm but $\leq$50 mm in greatest dimension
T3	Tumor > 50 mm in greatest dimension
T4	Tumor of any size with direct extension to the chest wall and/or to the skin (ulceration or macroscopic nodules); invasion of the dermis alone does not qualify as T4

pN category	pN criteria
pNX	Regional lymph nodes cannot be assessed (e.g., not removed for pathological study or previously removed)
pN0	No regional lymph node metastasis identified or ITCs only
pN0(i+)	ITCs only (malignant cell clusters no larger than 0.2 mm) in regional lymph node(s)
pN0(mol+)	Positive molecular findings by reverse transcriptase-polymerase chain reaction (RT-PCR); no isolated tumor cells (ITCs) detected
pN1	Micrometastases; or metastases in 1–3 axillary lymph nodes; and/or clinically negative internal mammary nodes with micrometastases or macrometastases by sentinel lymph node biopsy
pN1mi	Micrometastases (approximately 200 cells, larger than 0.2 mm, but none larger than 2.0 mm)
pN2	Metastases in four to nine axillary lymph nodes; or positive ipsilateral internal mammary lymph nodes by imaging in the absence of axillary lymph node metastases
pN3	Metastases in ten or more axillary lymph nodes;
	or in infraclavicular (Level III axillary) lymph nodes;
	or positive ipsilateral internal mammary lymph nodes by imaging in the presence of one or more positive Level I, II axillary lymph nodes;
	or in more than three axillary lymph nodes and micrometastases or macrometastases by sentinel lymph node biopsy in clinically negative ipsilateral internal mammary lymph nodes;
	or in ipsilateral supraclavicular lymph nodes

M category	M criteria
M0	No clinical or radiographic evidence of distant metastases
cM0(i+)	No clinical or radiographic evidence of distant metastases in the presence of tumor cells or deposits no larger than 0.2 mm detected microscopically or by molecular techniques in circulating blood, bone marrow, or other nonregional nodal tissue in a patient without symptoms or signs of metastases
cM1	Distant metastases detected by clinical and radiographic means
pM1	Any histologically proven metastases in distant organs; or if in non-regional nodes, metastases greater than 0.2 mm

Esophageal carcinoma pathologic staging

T category	T criteria
TX	Tumor cannot be assessed
T0	No evidence of primary tumor
Tis	High-grade dysplasia, defined as malignant cells confined to the epithelium by the basement membrane
T1	Tumor invades the lamina propria, muscularis mucosae, or submucosa
T2	Tumor invades the muscularis propria
T3	Tumor invades adventitia
T4	Tumor invades adjacent structures

N category	N criteria
NX	Regional lymph nodes cannot be assessed
N0	No regional lymph node metastasis
N1	Metastasis in one or two regional lymph nodes
N2	Metastasis in three to six regional lymph nodes
N3	Metastasis in seven or more regional lymph nodes

M category	M criteria
M0	No distant metastasis
M1	Distant metastasis

Gastric carcinoma pathologic staging

T category	T criteria
TX	Primary tumor cannot be assessed
T0	No evidence of primary tumor
Tis	Carcinoma in situ: intraepithelial tumor without invasion of the lamina propria, high-grade dysplasia
T1	Tumor invades the lamina propria, muscularis mucosae, or submucosa
T2	Tumor invades the muscularis propria
T3	Tumor penetrates the subserosal connective tissue without invasion of the visceral peritoneum or adjacent structures
T4	Tumor invades the serosa (visceral peritoneum) or adjacent structures

N category	N criteria
NX	Regional lymph node(s) cannot be assessed
N0	No regional lymph node metastasis
N1	Metastasis in one or two regional lymph nodes
N2	Metastasis in three to six regional lymph nodes
N3	Metastasis in seven or more regional lymph nodes

M category	M criteria
M0	No distant metastasis
M1	Distant metastasis

Gastrointestinal stromal tumors (GIST) staging

T category	T criteria
TX	Primary tumor cannot be assessed
T0	No evidence of primary tumor
T1	Tumor 2 cm or less
T2	Tumor more than 2 cm but not more than 5 cm
T3	Tumor more than 5 cm but not more than 10 cm
T4	Tumor more than 10 cm in greatest dimension

N category	N criteria
N0	No regional lymph node metastasis or unknown lymph node status
N1	Regional lymph node metastasis

M category	M criteria
M0	No distant metastasis
M1	Distant metastasis

Liver tumors pathologic staging

T category	T criteria
TX	Primary tumor cannot be assessed
T0	No evidence of primary tumor
T1	Solitary tumor ≤ 2 cm, or >2 cm without vascular invasion
T2	Solitary tumor > 2 cm *with* vascular invasion, or multiple tumors, none > 5 cm
T3	Multiple tumors, at least one of which is >5 cm
T4	Single tumor or multiple tumors of any size involving a major branch of the portal vein or hepatic vein, or tumor(s) with direct invasion of adjacent organs other than the gallbladder or with perforation of visceral peritoneum

N category	N criteria
NX	Regional lymph nodes cannot be assessed
N0	No regional lymph node metastasis
N1	Regional lymph node metastasis

M category	M criteria
M0	No distant metastasis
M1	Distant metastasis

Exocrine pancreas tumors pathologic staging

T category	T criteria
TX	Primary tumor cannot be assessed
T0	No evidence of primary tumor
Tis	Carcinoma in situ
	This includes high-grade pancreatic intraepithelial neoplasia (PanIn-3), intraductal papillary mucinous neoplasm with high-grade dysplasia, intraductal tubulopapillary neoplasm with high-grade dysplasia, and mucinous cystic neoplasm with high-grade dysplasia
T1	Tumor ≤ 2 cm in greatest dimension
T2	Tumor > 2 cm and ≤4 cm in greatest dimension
T3	Tumor > 4 cm in greatest dimension
T4	Tumor involves celiac axis, superior mesenteric artery, and/or common hepatic artery, regardless of size

N category	N criteria
NX	Regional lymph nodes cannot be assessed
N0	No regional lymph node metastases
N1	Metastasis in one to three regional lymph nodes
N2	Metastasis in four or more regional lymph nodes

M category	M criteria
M0	No distant metastasis
M1	Distant metastasis

Colorectal carcinoma pathologic staging

T category	T criteria
TX	Primary tumor cannot be assessed
T0	No evidence of primary tumor
Tis	Carcinoma in situ, intramucosal carcinoma (involvement of lamina propria with no extension through muscularis mucosae)
T1	Tumor invades the submucosa (through the muscularis mucosa but not into the muscularis propria)
T2	Tumor invades the muscularis propria
T3	Tumor invades through the muscularis propria into pericolorectal tissues
T4	Tumor invades the visceral peritoneum or invades or adheres to adjacent organ or structure

N category	N criteria
NX	Regional lymph nodes cannot be assessed
N0	No regional lymph node metastasis
N1	One to three regional lymph nodes are positive (tumor in lymph nodes measuring ≥ 0.2 mm), or any number of tumor deposits are present and all identifiable lymph nodes are negative
N2	Four or more regional nodes are positive

M category	M criteria
M0	No distant metastasis by imaging, and so on; no evidence of tumor in distant sites or organs (this category is not assigned by pathologists)
M1	Metastasis to one or more distant sites or organs or peritoneal metastasis is identified

Neuroendocrine tumors (NET) of the appendix pathologic staging

T category	T criteria
TX	Primary tumor cannot be assessed
T0	No evidence of primary tumor
T1	Tumor 2 cm or less in greatest dimension
T2	Tumor more than 2 cm but less than or equal to 4 cm

T category	T criteria
T3	Tumor more than 4 cm or with subserosal invasion or involvement of the mesoappendix
T4	Tumor perforates the peritoneum or directly invades other adjacent organs or structures (excluding direct mural extension to adjacent subserosa of adjacent bowel), for example, abdominal wall and skeletal muscle

N category	N criteria
NX	Regional lymph nodes cannot be assessed
N0	No regional lymph node metastasis
N1	Regional lymph node metastasis

M category	M criteria
M0	No distant metastasis
M1	Distant metastasis

Notes

Chromogranin A (CgA) is used as a biomarker for appendiceal NETs. CgA is a general NET
    marker that can reflect tumor load, monitor response to treatment, and correlate with a poor prognosis if elevated.

Other biomarkers, such as a plasma or urinary 5-hydroxyindoleacetic acid (5-HIAA) and serotonin, maybe used to identify patients with NETs of the gut or with carcinoid syndrome, but prospective trials are needed to validate their efficacy as a biomarker of appendiceal NETs.

CAUTION: CgA can be falsely elevated in the setting of proton-pump inhibitor use, chronic atrophic gastritis, renal failure, among others.

Ki-67 Proliferative Index

Histologic tumor grade is determined by Ki-67 proliferative index and/or the mitotic count. Ki-67 proliferative index is inversely correlated with patient prognosis.

Kidney tumors pathologic staging

T category	T criteria
TX	Primary tumor cannot be assessed
T0	No evidence of primary tumor
T1	Tumor ≤ 7 cm in greatest dimension, limited to the kidney
T2	Tumor > 7 cm in greatest dimension, limited to the kidney
T3	Tumor extends into major veins or perinephric tissues, but not into the ipsilateral adrenal gland and not beyond Gerota's fascia
T4	Tumor invades beyond Gerota's fascia (including contiguous extension into the ipsilateral adrenal gland)

N category	N criteria
NX	Regional lymph nodes cannot be assessed
N0	No regional lymph node metastasis
N1	Metastasis in regional lymph node(s)

M category	M criteria
M0	No distant metastasis
M1	Distant metastasis

Prostate cancer pathologic staging

T category	T criteria
T2	Organ confined
T3	Extraprostatic extension
T3a	Extra prostatic extension (unilateral or bilateral) or microscopic invasion of the bladder neck
T3b	Tumor invades seminal vesicle(s)
T4	Tumor is fixed or invades adjacent structures other than seminal vesicles such as external sphincter, rectum, bladder, levator muscles, and/or pelvic wall

N category	N criteria
NX	Regional lymph nodes cannot be assessed
N0	No positive regional nodes
N1	Metastases in regional node(s)

M category	M criteria
M0	No distant metastasis
M1	Distant metastasis
M1a	Nonregional lymph node(s)
M1b	Bone(s)
M1c	Other site(s) with or without bone disease

Note
There is *no* pathological T1 (pT1) category.

Testicular tumors pathologic staging

pT category	pT criteria
pTX	Primary tumor cannot be assessed
pT0	No evidence of primary tumor
pTis	Germ cell neoplasia in situ
pT1	Tumor limited to the testis (including rete testis invasion) without lymphovascular invasion
pT1a[a]	Tumor smaller than 3 cm in size
pT1b[a]	Tumor 3 cm or larger in size
pT2	Tumor limited to the testis (including rete testis invasion) with lymphovascular invasion
	OR
	Tumor invading hilar soft tissue or epididymis or penetrating visceral mesothelial layer covering the external surface of tunica albuginea with or without lymphovascular invasion
pT3	Tumor directly invades spermatic cord soft tissue with or without lymphovascular invasion
pT4	Tumor invades scrotum with or without lymphovascular invasion

pN category	pN criteria
pNX	Regional lymph nodes cannot be assessed
pN0	No regional lymph node metastasis
pN1	Metastasis with a lymph node mass 2 cm or smaller in greatest dimension and *less than or equal to five nodes positive*, none larger than 2 cm in greatest dimension
pN2	Metastasis with a lymph node mass larger than 2 cm but not larger than 5 cm in greatest dimension; or more than five nodes positive, none larger than 5 cm; or evidence of extranodal extension of tumor
pN3	Metastasis with a lymph node mass larger than 5 cm in greatest dimension

M category	M criteria
M0	No distant metastases
M1	Distant metastases
M1	Non-retroperitoneal nodal or pulmonary metastases
M1b	Non-pulmonary visceral metastases

[a]Subclassification of pT1 applies only to pure seminoma

Definition of serum markers (S)

S category	S criteria
SX	Marker studies not available or not performed
S0	Marker study levels within normal limits

S category	S criteria
S1	LDH < 1.5 × N* *and* hCG (mIU/mL) < 5000 *and* AFP (ng/mL) < 1000
S2	LDH 1.5–10 × N* *or* hCG (mIU/mL) 5000–50,000 *or* AFP (ng/mL) 1000–10,000
S3	LDH > 10 × N* *or* hCG (mIU/mL) > 50,000 *or* AFP (ng/mL) > 10,000

*N indicates the upper limit of normal for the LDH assay

Note
- Testicular cancer is one of the few malignancies in which serum tumor markers are incorporated in staging, as they can guide both diagnosis and management.
- These markers should be obtained at diagnosis, after orchiectomy, to monitor for response to treatment and relapse in patients on surveillance.

Uterine carcinoma pathologic staging

T category	FIGO stage	T criteria
TX		Primary tumor cannot be assessed
T0		No evidence of primary tumor
T1	I	Tumor confined to the corpus uteri, including endocervical glandular involvement
T1a	IA	Tumor limited to the endometrium or invading less than half the myometrium
T1b	IB	Tumor invading one half or more of the myometrium
T2	II	Tumor invading the stromal connective tissue of the cervix but not extending beyond the uterus. Does NOT include endocervical glandular involvement
T3	III	Tumor involving serosa, adnexa, vagina, or parametrium
T3a	IIIA	Tumor involving the serosa and/or adnexa (direct extension or metastasis)
T3b	IIIB	Vaginal involvement (direct extension or metastasis) or parametrial involvement
T4	IVA	Tumor invading the bladder mucosa and/or bowel mucosa (bullous edema is not sufficient to classify a tumor as T4)

N category	FIGO stage	N criteria
NX		Regional lymph nodes cannot be assessed
N0		No regional lymph node metastasis
N0(i+)		Isolated tumor cells in regional lymph node(s) no greater than 0.2 mm
N1	IIIC1	Regional lymph node metastasis to pelvic lymph nodes
N1mi	IIIC1	Regional lymph node metastasis (greater than 0.2 mm but not greater than 2.0 mm in diameter) to pelvic lymph nodes
N1a	IIIC1	Regional lymph node metastasis (greater than 2.0 mm in diameter) to pelvic lymph nodes

N category	FIGO stage	N criteria
N2	IIIC2	Regional lymph node metastasis to para-aortic lymph nodes, with or without positive pelvic lymph nodes
N2mi	IIIC2	Regional lymph node metastasis (greater than 0.2 mm but not greater than 2.0 mm in diameter) to para-aortic lymph nodes, with or without positive pelvic lymph nodes
N2a	IIIC2	Regional lymph node metastasis (greater than 2.0 mm in diameter) to para-aortic lymph nodes, with or without positive pelvic lymph nodes

M category	FIGO stage	M criteria
M0		No distant metastasis
M1	IVB	Distant metastasis (includes metastasis to inguinal lymph nodes, intraperitoneal disease, lung, liver, or bone)
		(It excludes metastasis to pelvic or para-aortic lymph nodes, vagina, uterine serosa, or adnexa)

The international Federation of Gynecology and Obstetrics (Fédération Internationale de Gynécologie et d'Obstétrique) (FIGO) system, uses surgical/pathological staging for corpus uteri cancer

The definitions of the T categories correspond to the stages accepted by FIGO

Further Reading

Amin MB, et al. AJCC cancer staging manual. Chicago: American College of Surgeons; 2018.

Surgical Margin Assessment

21

Ahmad Altaleb

Objective

- Learn how pathologists assess the surgical margin status, and the importance of local control of tumors.

One of the goals in the management of primary malignant tumors is complete surgical excision of the tumor with adequate margins of normal surrounding tissue to minimize the risk of local recurrence.

The optimal margin of normal tissue depends on many factors, including:

1. Anatomic location and preservation of function (the surgeon may have to settle for less than optimal margins when there are anatomic constraints, e.g., when tumors approach a major neurovascular structure).
2. Type of malignancy (nodular basal cell carcinomas and thin melanomas: a narrow margin of excision is adequate. A 2-cm margin is considered optimal for certain tumors such as soft tissue sarcomas, gastrointestinal stromal tumors(GIST), and low rectal carcinomas)
3. Tumor stage
4. Effectiveness of nonsurgical treatment modalities

When a resected specimen is submitted, the pathologist will decide how to take the section of the margin in relation to the tumor (Table 21.1 and Fig. 21.1). Next, when glass slides are ready, the pathologist would examine the margins microscopically to ascertain the margin status and measure the distance from the tumor edge to the inked surgical margin (Fig. 21.2). For example, in the case of infiltrating breast carcinoma, a positive margin is defined as ink on tumor cells (Fig. 21.3).

A. Altaleb (✉)
Histopathology Department, Mubarak Alkabeer Hospital, Jabriya, Kuwait

© The Editor(s) (if applicable) and The Author(s), under exclusive license to Springer Nature Switzerland AG 2021
A. Altaleb (ed.), *Surgical Pathology*,
https://doi.org/10.1007/978-3-030-53690-9_21

Table 21.1 Summary of the main methods for pathologic evaluation of surgical margins

Method	Comment
(A) Sections taken at *right angle/perpendicular* to the margin	– Used if tumor is macroscopically close to the margin – Can measure the distance from tumor cells to the margin by microscopic examination
(B) Sections taken *parallel* to the margin (*shave*)	– Used if tumor is macroscopically far away from the margin – Although it can tell if the margin is positive or negative, it cannot measure the distance from tumor cells to the margin by microscopic examination

Fig. 21.1 Schematic diagram of the main methods for pathologic evaluation of surgical margins. (**a**) Sections taken at right angles/perpendicular to the margin. (**b**) Sections taken parallel to the margin (shave)

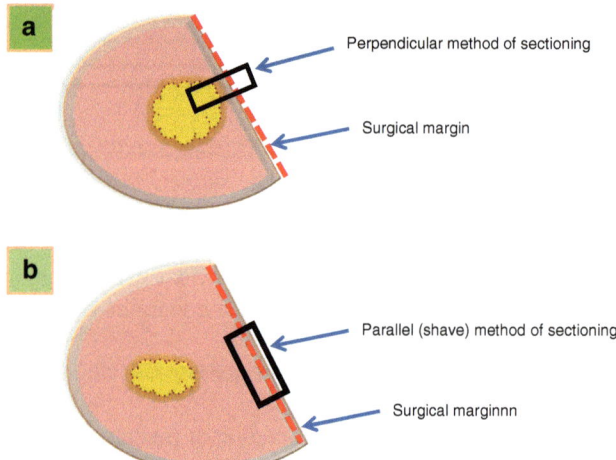

Fig. 21.2 Low power view of a breast carcinoma, which is far away from the margin (i.e., negative margin). The distance from the tumor edge to the margin is measured by microscopic examination

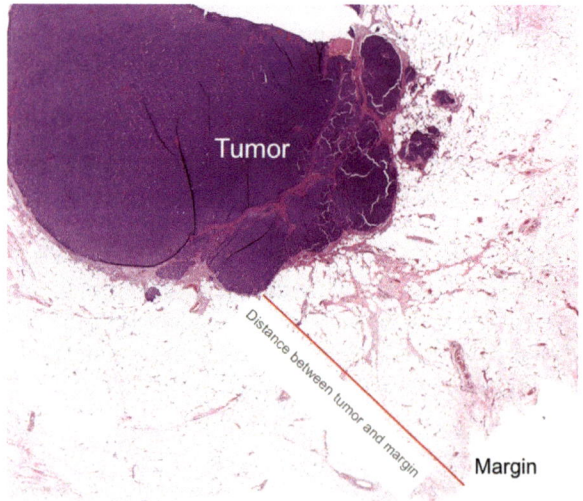

Fig. 21.3 High power magnification of an infiltrating breast carcinoma. Notice the black ink on tumor cells (i.e., positive margin)

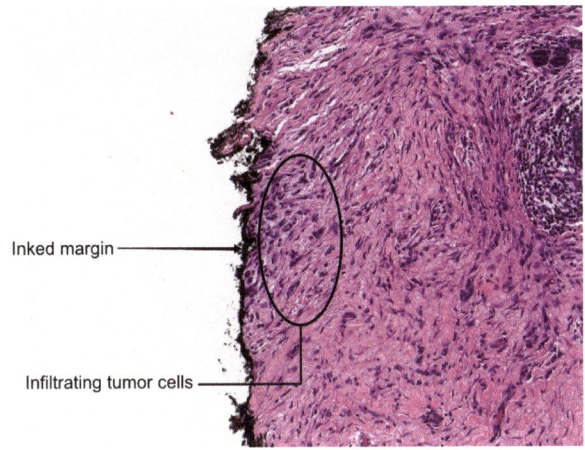

Inked margin

Infiltrating tumor cells

Clear or negative surgical margins reduce the risk of local recurrence of a tumor.

However, that will not guarantee that it will not recur. This could be explained by false-negative interpretation of the margins, tumor multifocality, or possibly the development of a new malignancy in a morphologically normal but genetically altered tissue.

Sometimes, if a margin is reported as positive, a subsequent re-excision specimen of that margin may not show any residual tumor. This may be attributed to:

1. The physically disruptive effects of surgery or
2. The biochemical inhibitory effects on tumor growth inherent in the healing process

Extent of Resection: A Rough Guide

The extent of resection largely depends on the organ involved and tumor type and its method of local spread (Fig. 21.4). In general, wide excision is the most efficacious method for local control and prevention of local recurrence (this is particularly valid for soft tissue sarcomas, certain cutaneous melanomas, and breast phyllodes tumors).

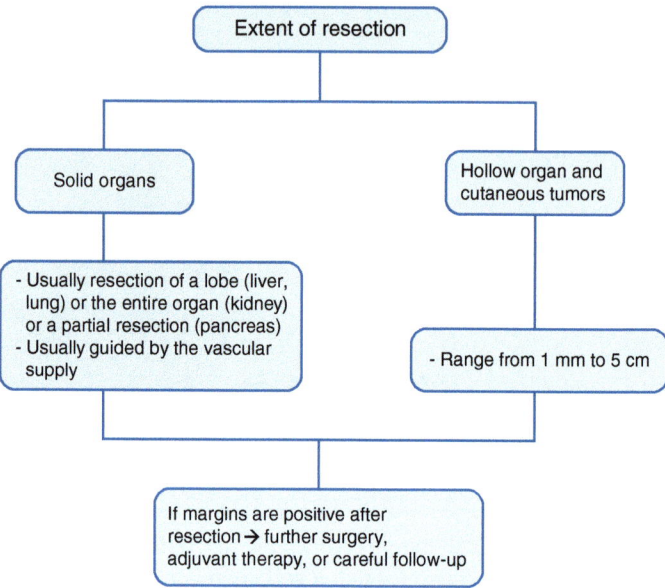

Fig. 21.4 Rough guide on the adequate extent of resection

Further Reading

Ramaswamy G. Washington manual of oncology. 2nd ed. Wolters Kluwer Medical: St. Louis; 2008.
Weidner N. Modern surgical pathology. Philadelphia: Saunders/Elsevier; 2009.

Metastases: A Visual Guide

22

Ahmad Altaleb

Objectives

- Learn the basic concepts of malignant tumor metastases, cancer of unknown primary (CUP) and the potential routs of distant metastases in different organs.
- Learn the patterns of lung metastases and their possible differential diagnoses.

High Yield Facts

Metastases

Malignant tumors can invade and destroy adjacent structures and spread to distant sites (metastasize) to cause death. See diagrams below, sites of distant metastases and patterns of metastases in the lung.

General Rules

- Carcinomas metastasize via lymphatics with some exceptions (e.g., follicular carcinoma of the thyroid, renal cell carcinoma, and choriocarcinoma)
- Sarcomas metastasize hematogenously with some exceptions (e.g., epithelioid sarcoma and synovial sarcoma)

Most common destination of distant metastases:

A. Altaleb (✉)
Histopathology Department, Mubarak Alkabeer Hospital, Jabriya, Kuwait

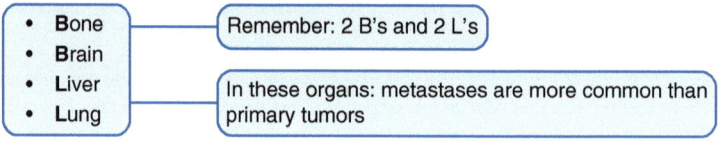

Cancer of Unknown Primary (CUP)

A malignant widespread metastatic disease without an identifiable primary site after extensive clinical investigations.

Accounts for 2.3–5% of new cancers.

Recently, a decline in the diagnosis of CUP owing to improvement in detection of primary tumor thus decreasing the unknown primaries.

Whole body (PET/CT) is the investigation of choice.

Heavy smokers and individuals with the lowest quartiles of waist circumference have a higher risk for developing CUP.

The site of origin may eventually be identified by pathologists (morphology and immunohistochemistry) or it may be found only at postmortem/autopsy examination.

Most common sites (if discovered)—pancreatobiliary, lung, and stomach.

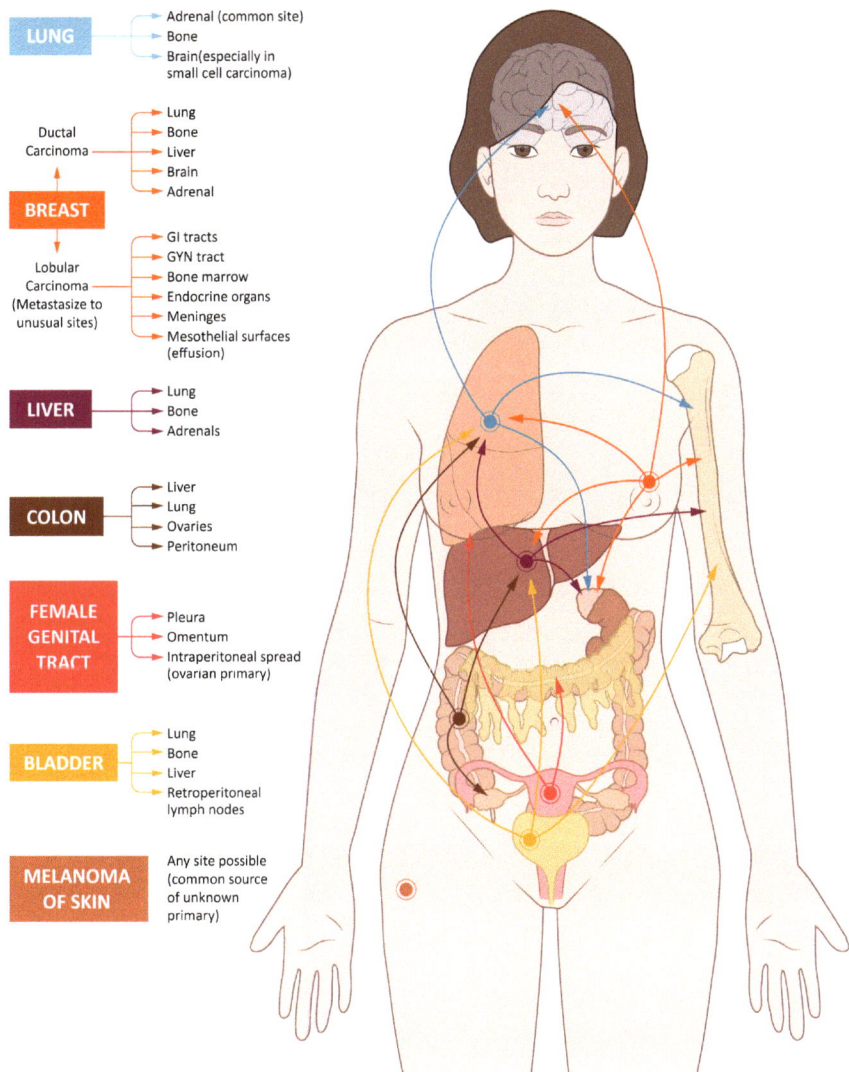

SITES OF DISTANT METASTASES
PART 1

LUNG
- Adrenal (common site)
- Bone
- Brain(especially in small cell carcinoma)

Ductal Carcinoma
- Lung
- Bone
- Liver
- Brain
- Adrenal

BREAST

Lobular Carcinoma (Metastasize to unusual sites)
- GI tracts
- GYN tract
- Bone marrow
- Endocrine organs
- Meninges
- Mesothelial surfaces (effusion)

LIVER
- Lung
- Bone
- Adrenals

COLON
- Liver
- Lung
- Ovaries
- Peritoneum

FEMALE GENITAL TRACT
- Pleura
- Omentum
- Intraperitoneal spread (ovarian primary)

BLADDER
- Lung
- Bone
- Liver
- Retroperitoneal lymph nodes

MELANOMA OF SKIN
Any site possible (common source of unknown primary)

Sites of distant metastases (primary site to distant location) – part 01

SITES OF DISTANT METASTASES
PART 2

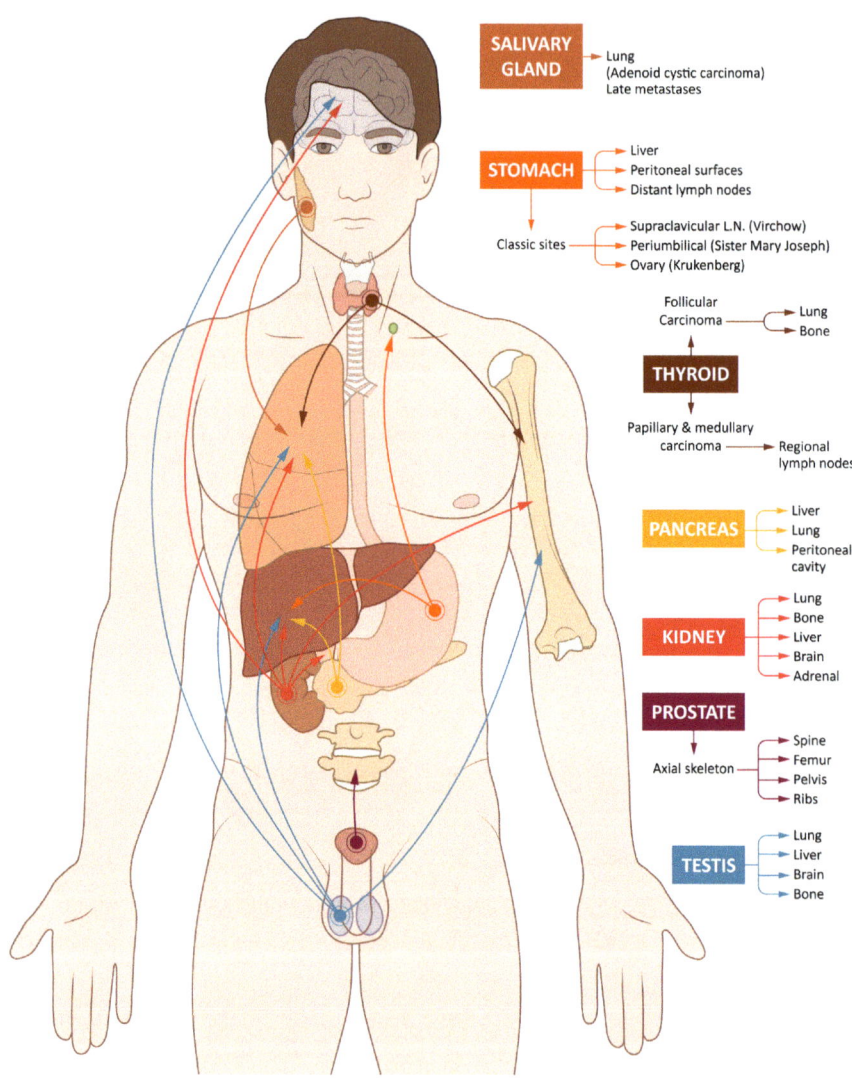

Sites of distant metastases (primary site to distant location) – part 02

PATTERNS OF METASTASES IN THE LUNG

1 **SOLITARY NODULE**

Classic Primary

Sarcoma
Endometrial
Melanoma
Colorectal
Germ cell tumor

Clinical DDX

Granuloma
Lung primary
Organizing
pneumonia

2 **PLEURAL SEEDING**

Classic Primary

Lung
Breast
Ovary

Clinical DDX

Mesothelioma

3 **MILIARY**
(usually associated with highly vascular tumors)

Classic Primary

Thyroid
Renal cell carcinoma

Clinical DDX

Tuberculosis
Carcinoid tumorlets

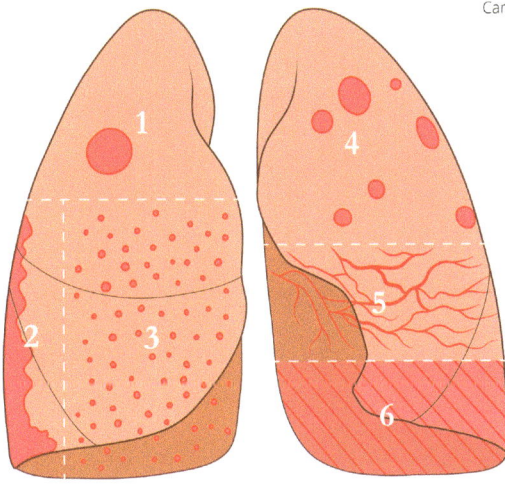

4 **MULTIPLE NODULES**
(most common pattern of metastases)

Classic Primary

Any

Clinical DDX

Granuloma
Organizing pneumonia
Abscess
Infarcts

5 **LYMPHANGITIC**

Classic Primary

Breast
Stomach
Pancreas
Lung
Prostate

Clinical DDX

Pulmonary edema
Infection
Interstitial lung disease

6 **CONSOLIDATIVE /
"PNEUMONIC-TYPE"**

Classic Primary

Invasive mucinous
adenocarcinoma
Pancreatobiliary

Clinical DDX

Pneumonia

Patterns of metastases in the lung (as detected by imaging)

Further Reading

Abbas AK, Aster JC, Kumar V. Robbins and Cotran pathologic basis of disease. Philadelphia: Elsevier/Saunders; 2015.

Qaseem A, Usman N, Jayaraj JS, Janapala RN, Kashif T. Cancer of unknown primary: a review on clinical guidelines in the development and targeted management of patients with the unknown primary site. Cureus. 2019;11(9):e5552.

Rekhtman N, Bishop JA. Quick reference handbook for surgical pathologists. Berlin: Springer; 2011.

Virtual Microscopy and Telepathology

Ahmad Altaleb

Objective

- Learn about the modern techniques in surgical pathology virtual slide sharing for the purpose of case consultation, education, and research among others.

A. Altaleb (✉)
Histopathology Department, Mubarak Alkabeer Hospital, Jabriya, Kuwait

VIRTUAL MICROSCOPY & TELEPATHOLOGY

Virtual Microscopy – A technique whereby glass slides are scanned and converted to digital/virtual slides which can then be viewed on a computer screen.

Telepathology – The practice whereby pathologists render diagnoses from distance by viewing electronic images.

✓ DIAGNOSTIC AND CLINICAL APPLICATIONS

"E-consultation"
- Review virtual slides anytime, anywhere
- No risk of losing tissue blocks or glass slides

Scanning selected cases for archiving
- Can be used in subsequent clinico-pathologic conferences
- Slide review available anytime in the record to guide any subsequent diagnostic workup

1° diagnosis
- In 2017 FDA cleared a digital pathology system to perform 1° diagnosis
- Many studies show same accuracy as 1° diagnosis by routine light microscopy, although it still requires extensive validation procedure
- Also? Cost/time saving issues

Quality assurance programs

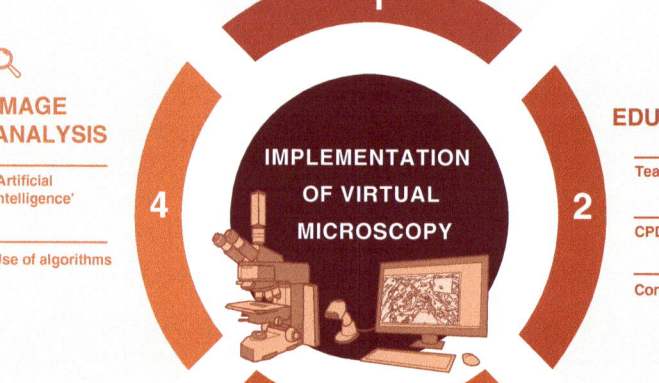

IMAGE ANALYSIS

'Artificial intelligence'

Use of algorithms

IMPLEMENTATION OF VIRTUAL MICROSCOPY

EDUCATION

Teaching

CPD Programs

Conferences

☀ RESEARCH

Image analysis

Tissue of patients enrolled in clinical trials

Consensus review of slides

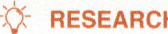

Electronic publishing of whole slides

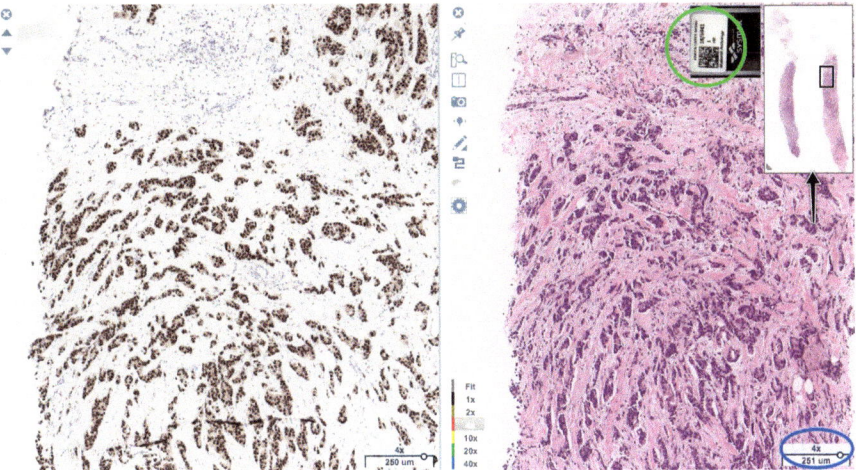

Fig. 23.1 Whole slide image viewer. Images of two juxtaposed hematoxylin and eosin (H&E) (right) and immunostained tissue sections (left). This method facilitates the matching of areas of interest and comparison of morphology and staining characteristics. Arrow: macroimage of the glass slide, green circle: label of the slide, and blue circle: scale bar

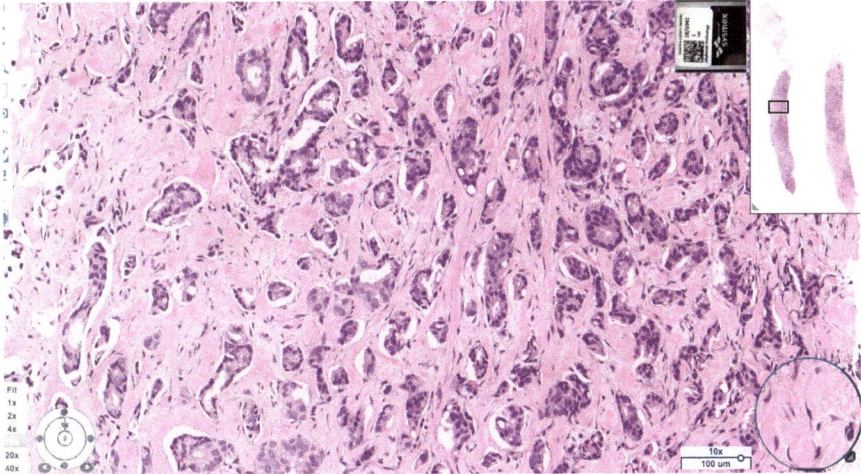

Fig. 23.2 A screen shot of a high-resolution hematoxylin and eosin (H&E) virtual slide image. Even at this medium power magnification, fine details of cytomorphology and tissue changes are seen clearly

Further Reading

Pfeifer JD, Humphrey PA, Ritter JH, Dehner LP. The Washington manual of surgical pathology. Philadelphia: Wolters Kluwer; 2019.

The Modern Pathologist Role at MDT Meeting

Ahmad Altaleb

Objective

- Learn about the vital role of pathologists as members in multidisciplinary team meetings and their contribution in patient management.

Multidisciplinary Team (MDT) Meeting

"A clinically focused meeting of health professionals that is involved in the management of patient treatment. This most commonly links to management of patients being considered with a diagnosis of malignancy (cancer MDT meeting)."

An effective MDT should include at least one pathologist. The classic role of the pathologist has been primarily to present pathology findings, such as resection specimens, biopsies, and cytology specimens. Presentation of the pathologic staging at tumor boards has been a particularly important role.

As the era of precision medicine is taking over, and as molecular testing finds more and more applicability in pathological diagnoses, the modern pathologists are increasingly playing an important supporting role in the determination of treatment recommendations by providing expert consultation on the use and interpretation of advanced molecular testing (Table 24.1).

Finally, it's important to emphasize that the health professionals' team members participating in MDT meetings have to maintain desirable behaviors and etiquette to achieve the maximum benefit of such meetings (Table 24.2).

A. Altaleb (✉)
Histopathology Department, Mubarak Alkabeer Hospital, Jabriya, Kuwait

© The Editor(s) (if applicable) and The Author(s), under exclusive license to Springer Nature Switzerland AG 2021
A. Altaleb (ed.), *Surgical Pathology*,
https://doi.org/10.1007/978-3-030-53690-9_24

Table 24.1 Summary of pathologist role at MDTs

Role of pathologist	Example
Diagnosis	– Tumor type, subtype/variant – Tumor grade
Pathologic staging	– pTNM (pathologic classification of anatomic extent of the malignancy)
Prognostic indicators assessment	– Grade of tumor – Lymphovascular invasion confirmation – Capsular invasion, e.g., thyroid follicular carcinoma – Tumor-infiltrating lymphocytes TILs, e.g., breast cancer – Tumor budding, e.g., colorectal cancer
Molecular testing and biomarkers assessment	– Testing for microsatellite instability status in colon cancer
Predictive markers assessment	– Breast cancer: ER, PR, and Her2 → for therapeutic decision making
Quality of cancer programs assessment	– Evaluation of mesorectal excision in rectal cancer

Table 24.2 Examples of expected team behavior/etiquette

Mutual respect among team members
An equal voice for all members
Different opinions valued
Ability to request and provide clarification if anything is unclear
Encouragement of constructive discussion/debate
Absence of personal agendas

Further Reading

Lowe J. The role of the lead pathologist and attending pathologists in the multidisciplinary team [Internet]. rcpath.org. 2014. https://www.rcpath.org/uploads/assets/bb9e7568-d41d-4d99-8ca12c8f0b67c8a5/170f47d9-7ec9-4f2f-bbe37d233cc93178/g087_roleofleadpathinmdt_mar2014.pdf.

Shakeel S, Mubarak M. Evolving and expanding role of pathologists in multidisciplinary team cancer care. J Coll Phys Surg Pak. 2018;28(1):3–4.

Washington K, Salaria SN. Expanding roles for pathologists as members of the multidisciplinary cancer care team [Internet]. Personalized medicine in oncology. 2016. [Cited 2020 Feb 26]. http://www.personalizedmedonc.com/publications/pmo/december-2016-vol-5-no-10/expanding-roles-for-pathologists-as-members-of-the-multidisciplinary-cancer-care-team/.

Part X

Errors in Surgical Pathology

Sources of Error in Surgical Pathology

Ahmad Altaleb

Objective

- Learn about the components of quality control in the surgical pathology laboratory and the potential errors in each component.

A. Altaleb (✉)
Histopathology Department, Mubarak Alkabeer Hospital, Jabriya, Kuwait

A. Altaleb (ed.), *Surgical Pathology*,
https://doi.org/10.1007/978-3-030-53690-9_25

SOURCES OF ERROR IN SURGICAL PATHOLOGY

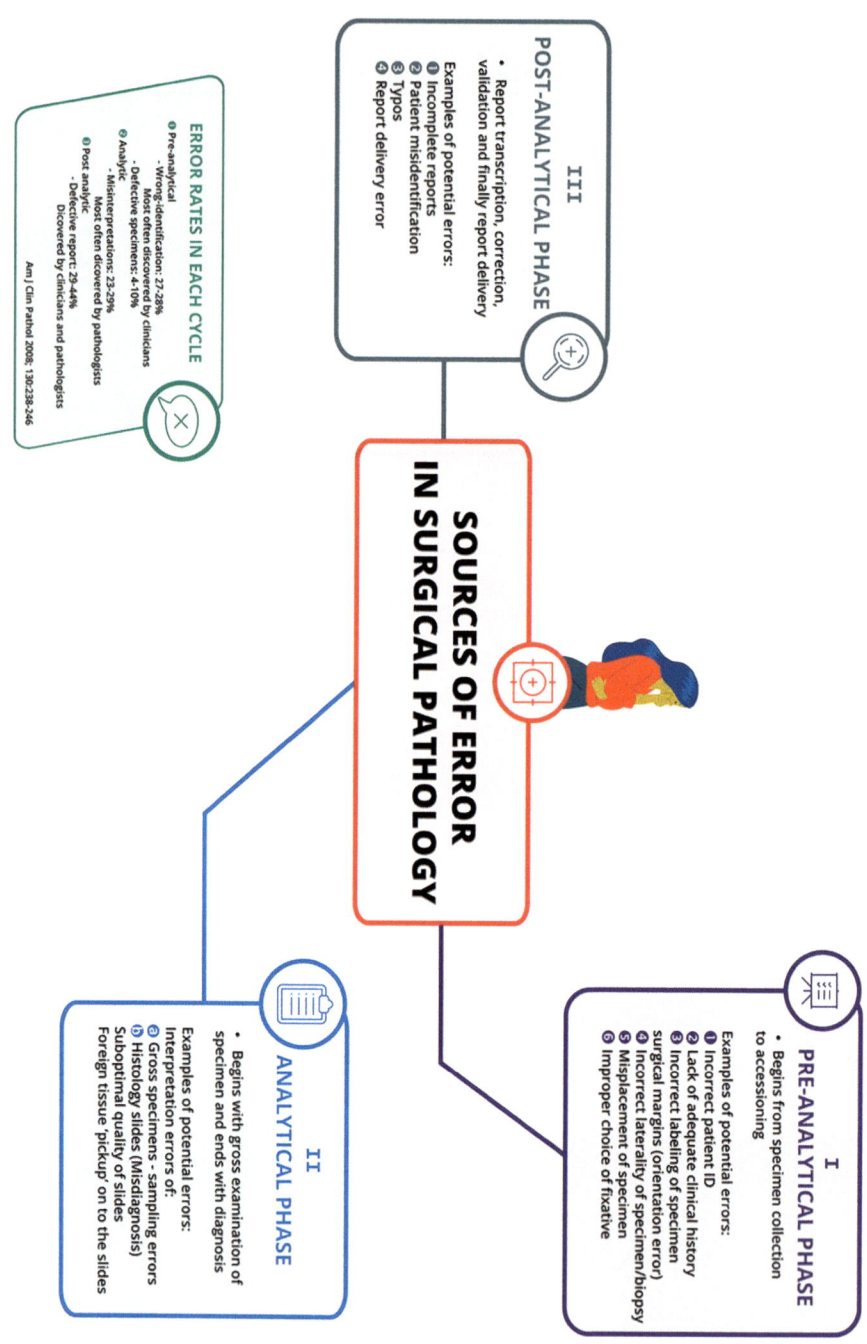

III POST-ANALYTICAL PHASE

- Report transcription, correction, validation and finally report delivery

Examples of potential errors:
1. Incomplete reports
2. Patient misidentification
3. Typos
4. Report delivery error

ERROR RATES IN EACH CYCLE

1. **Pre-analytical**
   - Wrong-identification: 27-28%
     Most often discovered by clinicians
   - Defective specimens: 4-10%
2. **Analytic**
   - Misinterpretations: 23-29%
     Most often discovered by pathologists
3. **Post analytic**
   - Defective report: 29-44%
     Dicovered by clinicians and pathologists

Am J Clin Pathol 2008; 130:238-246

I PRE-ANALYTICAL PHASE

- Begins from specimen collection to accessioning

Examples of potential errors:
1. Incorrect patient ID
2. Lack of adequate clinical history
3. Incorrect labeling of specimen
4. Incorrect margins (orientation error)
5. Incorrect laterality of specimen/biopsy
6. Misplacement of specimen
7. Improper choice of fixative

II ANALYTICAL PHASE

- Begins with gross examination of specimen and ends with diagnosis

Examples of potential errors:
Interpretation errors of:
1. Gross specimens - sampling errors
2. Histology slides (Misdiagnosis)
   Suboptimal quality of slides
   Foreign tissue 'pickup' on to the slides

Further Reading

Pfeifer JD, Humphrey PA, Ritter JH, Dehner LP. The Washington manual of surgical pathology. Philadelphia: Wolters Kluwer; 2019.

Quality Control and Assurance in Anatomic Pathology: The Moffitt Experience [Internet]. moffitt.org. 2012. [Cited 2019]. https://moffitt.org/media/6067/centeno-qc-and-qa-in-anatomic-pathology.pdf.

Santana MF, Ferreira LCde L. Errors in Surgical Pathology Laboratory [Internet]. IntechOpen. IntechOpen; 2018 [cited 2020Aug1]. Available from: https://www.intechopen.com/books/quality-control-in-laboratory/errors-in-surgical-pathology-laboratory

Index